Enhanced Recovery After Surgery: Past, Present and Future

Editor

DANIEL I. CHU

SURGICAL CLINICS
OF NORTH AMERICA

www.surgical.theclinics.com

Consulting Editor
RONALD F. MARTIN

December 2018 • Volume 98 • Number 6

ELSEVIER

1600 John F. Kennedy Boulevard • Suite 1800 • Philadelphia, Pennsylvania, 19103-2899

http://www.surgical.theclinics.com

SURGICAL CLINICS OF NORTH AMERICA Volume 98, Number 6
December 2018 ISSN 0039-6109, ISBN-13: 978-0-323-64212-5

Editor: John Vassallo, j.vassallo@elsevier.com
Developmental Editor: Meredith Madeira

Surgical Clinics of North America (ISSN 0039-6109) is published bimonthly by Elsevier Inc., 360 Park Avenue South, New York, NY 10010-1710. Months of publication are February, April, June, August, October, and December. Business and Editorial Offices: 1600 John F. Kennedy Blvd., Suite 1800, Philadelphia, PA 19103-2899. Periodicals postage paid at New York, NY and additional mailing offices. Subscription prices are $350.00 per year for US individuals, $802.00 per year for US institutions, $100.00 per year for US students and residents, $420.00 per year for Canadian individuals, $1015.00 per year for Canadian institutions, $475.00 for international individuals, $1015.00 per year for international institutions and $225.00 per year for Canadian and foreign students/residents. To receive student/resident rate, orders must be accompanied by name of affiliated institution, date of term, and the *signature* of program/residency coordinator on institution letterhead. Orders will be billed at individual rate until proof of status is received. Foreign air speed delivery is included in all *Clinics* subscription prices. All prices are subject to change without notice. POSTMASTER: Send address changes to *Surgical Clinics*, Elsevier Health Sciences Division, Subscription Customer Service, 3251 Riverport Lane, Maryland Heights, MO 63043. **Customer Service (orders, claims, online, change of address): Telephone: 1-800-654-2452 (U.S. and Canada); 314-447-8871 (outside U.S. and Canada). Fax: 314-447-8029. E-mail: journalscustomerservice-usa@elsevier.com (for print support); journalsonline support-usa@elsevier.com (for online support).**

Reprints. For copies of 100 or more, of articles in this publication, please contact the Commercial Reprints Department, Elsevier Inc., 360 Park Avenue South, New York, New York 10010-1710. Tel. 212-633-3874, Fax: 212-633-3820, E-mail: reprints@elsevier.com.

The Surgical Clinics of North America is also published in Spanish by McGraw-Hill Interamericana Editores S.A., P.O. Box 5-237 06500 Mexico D.F. Mexico; and in Portuguese by Interlivros Edicoes Ltda., Rua Comandante Coelho 1085, CEP 21250, Rio de Janeiro, Brazil; and in Greek by Paschalidis Medical Publications, Athens Greece.

The Surgical Clinics of North America is covered in *MEDLINE/PubMed (Index Medicus), EMBASE/Excerpta Medica, Current Contents/Clinical Medicine, Current Contents/Life Sciences, Science Citation Index,* and *ISI/BIOMED.*

Contributors

CONSULTING EDITOR

RONALD F. MARTIN, MD, FACS
Colonel (ret.), United States Army Reserve, Chair, Department of Surgery, York Hospital,
York, Maine, USA

EDITOR

DANIEL I. CHU, MD, FACS, FASCRS
Associate Professor, Division of Gastrointestinal Surgery, Department of Surgery, The
University of Alabama at Birmingham, Birmingham, Alabama, USA

AUTHORS

THOMAS A. ALOIA, MD
Department of Surgical Oncology, The University of Texas MD Anderson Cancer Center,
Houston, Texas, USA

GABRIELE BALDINI, MD, MSc
Department of Anesthesia, McGill University Health Centre, Montreal, Québec,
Canada

JAI BIKHCHANDANI, MD
St Elizabeth Physicians, Department of Surgery, St Elizabeth Hospital, Edgewood,
Kentucky, USA

DARAN BROWN, MBA, RN
Manager, Department of Quality and Patient Safety, UAB Hospital, Birmingham, Alabama,
USA

FRANCESCO CARLI, MD, MPhil
Department of Anesthesia, McGill University Health Centre, Montreal, Québec, Canada

DANIEL I. CHU, MD, FACS, FASCRS
Associate Professor, Division of Gastrointestinal Surgery, Department of Surgery, The
University of Alabama at Birmingham, Birmingham, Alabama, USA

JEFFREY B. DOBYNS, DO, MSHA, CMQ
Associate Professor of Anesthesiology and Perioperative Medicine, Associate Medical
Director of Preoperative Assessment, Consultation, and Treatment Clinic, The University
of Alabama at Birmingham School of Medicine, Birmingham, Alabama, USA

W. JONATHAN DUNKMAN, MD
Assistant Professor, Department of Anesthesiology, Duke University, Duke University
Medical Center, Durham, North Carolina, USA

LIANE S. FELDMAN, MD
Professor of Surgery, Chief, Division of General Surgery, McGill University Health Centre, Steinberg-Bernstein Centre for Minimally Invasive Surgery and Innovation, Montreal, Québec, Canada

VANESSA FERREIRA, MSc
Department of Anesthesia, McGill University Health Centre, Department of Kinesiology and Physical Education, McGill University, Montreal, Québec, Canada

AMANDA HAYMAN, MD, MPH
Colon and Rectal Surgeon, Division of Gastrointestinal and Minimally Invasive Surgery, The Oregon Clinic, Affiliate Assistant Professor, Department of Surgery, Oregon Health & Science University, Portland, Oregon, USA

DAVID W. LARSON, MD, MBA
Division of Colon and Rectal Surgery, Mayo Clinic, Rochester, Minnesota, USA

CHARLES A. LEATH III, MD, MSPH, FACS
Professor, Division of Gynecologic Oncology, Department of Obstetrics and Gynecology, The University of Alabama at Birmingham, Birmingham, Alabama, USA

LAWRENCE LEE, MD, PhD
Assistant Professor of Surgery, McGill University Health Centre, Steinberg-Bernstein Centre for Minimally Invasive Surgery and Innovation, Montreal, Québec, Canada

HEATHER A. LILLEMOE, MD
Department of Surgical Oncology, The University of Texas MD Anderson Cancer Center, Houston, Texas, USA

DAVID LISKA, MD, FACS, FASCRS
Assistant Professor of Surgery, Department of Colorectal Surgery, Digestive Disease and Surgery Institute, Cleveland Clinic, Cleveland, Ohio, USA

JESSICA Y. LIU, MD, MS
Clinical Scholar in Residence, American College of Surgeons, Division of Research and Optimal Patient Care, Chicago, Illinois, USA; General Surgery Resident, Department of Surgery, Emory University, Atlanta, Georgia, USA

MICHAEL W. MANNING, MD, PhD
Assistant Professor, Department of Anesthesiology, Duke University, Duke University Medical Center, Durham, North Carolina, USA

ISABEL C. MARQUES, MD
Department of Surgery, The University of Alabama at Birmingham, Birmingham, Alabama, USA

ROBIN S. McLEOD, MD, FRCSC, FACS
Vice Chair, Quality and Best Practices, Department of Surgery, University of Toronto, Vice President, Clinical Programs and Quality Initiatives, Cancer Care Ontario, Toronto, Ontario, Canada

AMIT MERCHEA, MD
Division of Colon and Rectal Surgery, Mayo Clinic, Assistant Professor of Surgery, Mayo Clinic College of Medicine, Jacksonville, Florida, USA

JEFFREY WELLS NIX, MD
Assistant Professor, Department Urology, The University of Alabama at Birmingham, Birmingham, Alabama, USA

JUHAN PAISTE, MD, MBA
Vice Chair and Executive Medical Director of Anesthesia Services, Associate Professor, Department of Anesthesiology and Perioperative Medicine, The University of Alabama at Birmingham School of Medicine, Birmingham, Alabama, USA

EMILY A. PEARSALL, MSc
Manager, Best Practice in Surgery, Department of Surgery, University of Toronto, Toronto, Ontario, Canada

AVA SAIDIAN, MD
Resident Physician, Department Urology, The University of Alabama at Birmingham, Birmingham, Alabama, USA

JEFFREY W. SIMMONS, MD
Co-Director of Colorectal Enhanced Recovery After Surgery Program, Medical Director of Preoperative Assessment, Consultation, and Treatment Clinic, Associate Professor, Department of Anesthesiology and Perioperative Medicine, The University of Alabama at Birmingham School of Medicine, Birmingham, Alabama, USA

HALLER J. SMITH, MD
Fellow/Clinical Instructor, Division of Gynecologic Oncology, Department of Obstetrics and Gynecology, The University of Alabama at Birmingham, Birmingham, Alabama, USA

JOHN MICHAEL STRAUGHN Jr, MD
Professor, Division of Gynecologic Oncology, Department of Obstetrics and Gynecology, The University of Alabama at Birmingham, Birmingham, Alabama, USA

JULIE THACKER, MD, FACS, FASCRS
Associate Professor of Surgery, Duke University, Durham, North Carolina, USA

JIM P. TIERNAN, MD, PhD, FRCS
Fellow, Department of Colorectal Surgery, Digestive Disease and Surgery Institute, Cleveland Clinic, Cleveland, Ohio, USA

TYLER S. WAHL, MD, MSPH
Department of Surgery, The University of Alabama at Birmingham, Birmingham, Alabama, USA

ELIZABETH C. WICK, MD
Associate Professor of Surgery, Division of General Surgery, University of California, San Francisco, San Francisco, California, USA

ANISA XHAJA, MHA, MSHQS
Manager of Quality Improvement, Quality, Patient Safety and Clinical Effectiveness, UAB Hospital, Birmingham, Alabama, USA

JEFFREY V. WELCH, MD
Assistant Professor, Department [Surgery], The University of Alabama at Birmingham, Birmingham, Alabama, USA

BRIAN PAPPETT, MD, MBA
Vice Chief and Executive Medical Director of Anesthesia Services, Department of Anesthesiology and Perioperative Medicine, The University of Alabama at Birmingham School of Medicine, Birmingham, Alabama, USA

EMILY A. PEARSALL, MSc
Manager, Best Practice in Surgery, Department of Surgery, University of Toronto, Toronto, Ontario, Canada

ANA GRIJALVA, MD
Resident Physician, Department [Biology], The University of Alabama at Birmingham, Birmingham, Alabama, USA

JEFFREY W. SIMMONS, MD
Co-Director of Cardiac [Critical Care], Resident Affairs, Fellowship Program, Medical Director of Perioperative Assessment, Consultation, and Treatment Clinic, Associate Professor, Department of Anesthesiology and Perioperative Medicine, The University of Alabama at Birmingham School of Medicine, Birmingham, Alabama, USA

HALLEY J. SMITH, MD
Fellow, Medical Instructor, Division of Gynecologic Oncology, Department of Obstetrics and Gynecology, The University of Alabama at Birmingham, Birmingham, Alabama, USA

JOHN MICHAEL STRAUGHN Jr., MD
Professor, Division of Gynecologic Oncology, Department of Obstetrics and Gynecology, The University of Alabama at Birmingham, Birmingham, Alabama, USA

JULIE THACKER, MD, FACS, FASCRS
Associate Professor of Surgery, Duke University, Durham, North Carolina, USA

JIM F. TIERNAN, MD, PhD, FACS
Fellow, Department of Colorectal Surgery, Digestive Disease and Surgery Institute, Cleveland Clinic, Cleveland, Ohio, USA

TYLER S. WAHL, MD, MSPH
Department of Surgery, The University of Alabama at Birmingham, Birmingham, Alabama, USA

ELIZABETH C. WICK, MD
Associate Professor of Surgery, Quality Officer, Department of Surgery, University of California San Francisco, San Francisco, California, USA

APRIL ZEHM, MD, MSHPC
Assistant Professor, Hematology/Oncology and Palliative Care, Medical College of Wisconsin, Milwaukee, Wisconsin, USA

Contents

Enhanced Recovery is broadly defined as the application of evidence based perioperative care elements for improved surgical outcomes. Demonstration of decreasing surgical stress with innovation of surgical technique, in combination with pressure to drive down health care costs, have coalesced into a unique version of perioperative medicine in the United States. The US government has failed to show interest; there are no performance metrics, no participation requirements, and certainly no monetary incentives for implementation of best perioperative practices. When considering the term, Enhanced Recovery is, in its broadest sense, an amalgam of industry, innovation, patient-focused care, cost-effective strategies, and collaboration with a goal of best perioperative outcomes.

Enhanced recovery after surgery (ERAS) is an evidence-based protocol that aims to decrease the physiologic stress response to surgery and maintain postoperative physiologic function. This best practice bundle plays a significant role in improving surgical quality by impacting important quality metrics such as length of stay, hospital-acquired infections, readmissions, and patient experience. Adherence to ERAS as a collective bundle is more important than individual components in improving quality metrics, and this can only be achieved with data-driven information through auditing and interdisciplinary collaboration.

Enhanced recovery programs were developed as a means for improving patient recovery after surgery with a multifaceted approach including several interventions in the perioperative period. There is now sufficient evidence in the literature that enhanced recovery programs have actually shortened hospital length of stay after colorectal surgery. Nonetheless, the impact of these successful programs on patient-reported outcomes like functional recovery and return to baseline quality of life is not known.

Value in health care is defined as the best outcome that matters to the patient at the lowest cost. Therefore, a valuable intervention is one that either results in better outcomes at the same cost, the same outcomes at lower cost, or in the best-case scenario, better outcomes at lower cost. Enhanced recovery pathways (ERPs) increase value by improving clinical outcomes without increasing costs. ERPs do not increase overall costs, even when implementation and maintenance costs are considered. More research on patient-reported outcomes and other downstream effects of ERPs is required to fully characterize their true value.

Preoperative risk assessment is valuable only if subsequent targeted optimization of patient care is allowed. Early assessment of high-risk surgical patients is essential to facilitate appropriate optimization. Preoperative assessment and optimization should not be exclusively focused on patients' comorbidities, but also include nutritional assessment, functional capacity, and promote healthy life style habits that affect surgical outcomes (eg, smoking cessation); it requires a multidisciplinary approach.

Enhanced recovery after surgery is an evidence-based, multimodal approach to the perioperative care of a patient undergoing surgery. These pathways seek to attenuate the stress response to surgery facilitating postoperative recovery. Analgesia is a critical component of these pathways, because optimal pain relief is critical for patients to mobilize quickly after surgery, preventing such complications as infection and thromboembolism. Traditional analgesic regimens for major surgery rely heavily on opioids to provide analgesia but can cause a wide range of serious side effects, delaying recovery. Enhanced recovery protocols should incorporate multimodal analgesic strategies that minimize opioid use and optimize analgesia.

Ideal fluid management is a critical component of enhanced recovery after surgery protocols and should be considered throughout the perioperative period. The goal of preoperative fluid management is for the patient to arrive to the operating room euvolemic. Intraoperative goals of fluid management are to preserve intravascular volume and minimize salt and water uptake through intravenous crystalloid infusions. Postoperatively, once patients are tolerant of oral fluid intake, intravenous fluids are not required and should be restarted only if clinically necessary. This article reviews evidence-based, best practices for intraoperative fluid management for patients undergoing surgery within an enhanced recovery after surgery pathway.

Numerous reports have documented the effectiveness of Enhanced Recovery after Surgery (ERAS) pathways in improving recovery and decreasing morbidity and length of stay. However, there is also increasing evidence that ERAS guidelines are difficult to adopt and require the commitment of all members of the perioperative team. Multiple barriers related to limited hospital resources (financial, staffing, space restrictions, and education), active or passive resistance from members of the perioperative team, and lack of data and/or education have been identified. Thus, ERAS® guidelines require a tailored implementation strategy to increase adherence.

A growing body of evidence suggests that the implementation of an enhanced recovery after surgery (ERAS) clinical pathway can accelerate recovery and reduce length of stay through the use of a multimodal program that includes guidelines for optimal pain relief, stress reduction, early nutrition, and early mobilization. The article discusses the importance of the nursing body in improving institutional compliance to ERAS clinical pathway measures and describes specific nursing barriers observed in the ERAS implementation in an academic medical center.

Surgical disparities exist. Certain surgical populations suffer from disproportionately worse access, care, and outcomes in surgery. Opportunities exist to better identify, understand, and reduce these disparities. Enhanced Recovery After Surgery (ERAS) pathways use standardized perioperative processes and a multidisciplinary philosophy to deliver best-evidence surgical care to *all* patients. As a result, ERAS provides a uniquely pragmatic model for improving outcomes and reducing disparities in vulnerable surgical populations. The value of ERAS may therefore extend beyond its traditional benefits to the even greater pursuit of health equity.

Multidisciplinary collaboration and administrative support are essential to enhanced recovery program (ERP) success. The key tenets for ERP are opiate-sparing pain regimen, decreased fasting, and minimizing intravenous fluids. Getting buy-in from community surgeons may be difficult due to varied practice patterns and clinical fragmentation. Prospective tracking of ERP outcomes will allow for more targeted interventions.

Jim P. Tiernan and David Liska

Enhanced recovery after surgery (ERAS) has been established as a safe and effective tool for early recovery and discharge after colorectal resection. This article reviews the latest additions and refinements to ERAS protocols and also examines those interventions that seem to have limited clinical benefit for colorectal patients.

Heather A. Lillemoe and Thomas A. Aloia

Enhanced recovery after surgery (ERAS) pathways target specific areas within perioperative patient care in a multidisciplinary and evidence-based manner. Because of the subsequent positive outcomes associated with its use, ERAS has expanded to most surgical subspecialties, including hepatopancreatobiliary surgery. Although certain concepts are universal to all ERAS protocols, there are unique areas of emphasis pertaining to the hepatopancreatobiliary specialties, which will be highlighted throughout this article. In addition, some of the less frequently discussed aspects of enhanced recovery, including patient-reported outcomes, recovery assessment, cost, and auditing, will be addressed.

Ava Saidian and Jeffrey Wells Nix

Enhanced recovery after surgery programs were developed as a type of standardized evidence-based perioperative care protocols. The necessity and benefit of clinical care pathways is not a new phenomenon in urology and have been a big part of the evolution of care for urology patients, especially in terms of urologic oncology. This article discusses the key components of evidence-based perioperative care in key urologic procedures. These protocols have been shown to decrease length of stay, decrease complications, and reduce cost.

Haller J. Smith, Charles A. Leath III, and John Michael Straughn Jr

Many of the enhanced recovery after surgery principles initially developed for colorectal surgery can be successfully applied to gynecologic oncology and lead to significant improvements in perioperative care. Enhanced recovery after surgery guidelines specific to gynecologic oncology were published in 2016 and provide a framework for the development and implementation of institutional protocols. Identification of key stakeholders and a multidisciplinary approach are critical to identifying which principles are best suited for implementation at a particular institution and for ensuring success of the protocol. Herein, we review our experience with protocol development and implementation on a gynecologic oncology service.

Although the utilization of enhanced recovery after surgery (ERAS) pathways has become more prevalent, issues of compliance and implementation remain. Limiting the complexity of new ERAS protocols by maintaining the core elements of ERAS, along with the development of complementary protocols (prehabilitation, the perioperative surgical home, and telemedicine) may improve overall uptake and subsequent patient outcomes. The future directions of ERAS should be centered on improving the dissemination of the practice and ongoing expansion of patient care outside the immediate hospital period.

SURGICAL CLINICS
OF NORTH AMERICA

SERIES OF RELATED INTEREST

Advances in Surgery
Available at: www.advancessurgery.com
Surgical Oncology Clinics
Available at: www.surgonc.theclinics.com
Thoracic Surgery Clinics
Available at: www.thoracic.theclinics.com

THE CLINICS ARE AVAILABLE ONLINE!
Access your subscription at:
www.theclinics.com

Foreword

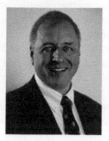

Ronald F. Martin, MD, FACS
Consulting Editor

Someone once told me that when she was little she thought her parents knew everything; then when she was a teenager, she was convinced her parents knew nothing. She went on to say that after she moved on and a got a place of her own, she was astounded by how much her parents had learned. We all seem to go through arcs of understanding and awareness. When most of us are learning something, we begin by realizing that we don't know much; then we progress to thinking we have a pretty good understanding, and then, as we study even more, we (usually) progress to realizing we don't know as much as we thought we did.

As I started learning medicine, we as a nation were entering a time when we began to look at the medical workplace in terms of "markets." The idea of taking care of patients one at a time without regard to economics was dying quickly. At first, the discussion was about cost-awareness and cost-containment, but over several years, the lingo started to shift to covered-lives and "per member per year" costs.

Various people with very serious slide presentations—later replaced by Power Point—gave elegant prognostications about how we would all shift form "phase 1" to "phase 4" markets. It was predicted that as market forces evolved, doctors/hospitals would be paying for everyone's health care costs out of some allotted fund for global coverage. Providing entities would progress from assuming no risk of cost to sharing risk of cost to owning all the risk of cost. Countless hours were spent in boardrooms—it was as if Congress had passed a "full employment for consultants" act.

Some of the information we were given was actually helpful, especially if one had never really thought of the "system" as an actual system. Some of the information was horrible as the guesses and warnings evaporated on contact with reality. Nonetheless, through all the smoke and mirrors, through all the "Toyota" lectures and "lean six sigma" presentations, one element seemed impervious to rebuttal: there was not nor was there going to be enough resources to do everything for everybody in all circumstances. We were going to have to make economic decisions. We would have to ration...somehow.

At the beginning, this seemed unfathomable, if not antithetical to our oaths to care for patients. However, as time went by and we studied the problem, I began to think

Surg Clin N Am 98 (2018) xiii–xv
https://doi.org/10.1016/j.suc.2018.09.012
0039-6109/18/© 2018 Published by Elsevier Inc.

surgical.theclinics.com

I had an answer or at least a start of an answer to mitigate the competing interests. It didn't matter whether one worked in a phase 1, total fee-for-service market, or a phase 4, globally compensated for all services population market. The answer was you just had to be better, faster, and cheaper at providing care. Either better, faster, and cheaper than you had been or at least better, faster, and cheaper than your competitors were. Economics and risk taking put aside, increased efficiencies would allow us to remain competitive and to survive in an economy that was determined to bend the cost curve downward without compromising patient care. It was a revelation to me. It was an idea that was stunningly simple, and it was bulletproof.

And it was dead wrong.

It is actually wrong for lots of reasons. Even if efficiencies were as deliverable as we would like them to be, future increased demand offsets any incremental gains from efficiency. Technology and electronic health records did not deliver on promises of greater throughput at less cost. Even more contributing to the efficiency fallacy is that the US health care market, while being somewhat self-contained, still has a great deal of interaction with other economies, which further complicates matters. However, the greatest reason to doubt that improving efficiency would reduce cost is that it would most likely run contrary to some very powerful interests.

To paraphrase, it is difficult to get someone to understand something when his/her salary is dependent on not understanding that "something." The "cost" we pay for our health care is roughly equal to the salary of everybody who either works or provides goods and services to that system plus the profits that are taken out. The willingness to reduce cost depends on how the savings are to be distributed. And therein lies the rub. From an economic perspective, being better, faster, and cheaper is most desirable when the one who creates the economic efficiency derives the economic benefit. Our health care system rarely works quite that way. Every sector of the health care market has needs and reason to protect its revenue stream.

For practitioners of surgery and medicine, there are other than economic benefits to be considered as we care for those who are afflicted. Our patients' well-being is a very real benefit. Particularly for those of us who operate on patients, anything we can do to make their process less painful, complicated, or disruptive of their lives is of tremendous value. The professional goal to develop and implement ways to "enhance recovery after surgery" has been absolutely directed to this end. (Parenthetically, the use of the term "enhanced recovery after surgery" in this issue is used as a generic term. In any instance where the term is used in a proprietary sense, we have made a concerted effort to recognize it specifically as such.)

We all share a professional goal to minimize the adverse impact of surgical treatment on patients. We all should try to relieve suffering of both a physical and an economic nature whenever and however we can. Dr Chu and his colleagues have provided us with a comprehensive review of processes and information to help us help our patients better prepare for and better recover from operations. It should improve patient health and also improve the value of the service to the patient by reducing unnecessary cost. We are deeply grateful to all of our contributors to this issue for their excellent work.

As I continue to try to understand what we do and why we do it, I realize how much more I don't know. We live and work in a complex system in even more complex times. I remain skeptical about how we will all overcome forces that impede our progress but endeavor to not become cynical. I remain optimistic that the arc of our progress will bend toward doing the right thing for our patients and for our communities. If ever I doubt that, I remind myself of the hundreds of colleagues we all have who have contributed to this series in a most selfless way. I think there are more people who wish to be part of the solution than who wish to be part of the problem. If I am correct, then we have good reason for hope.

Ronald F. Martin, MD, FACS, Colonel (ret.)
United States Army Reserve
Department of Surgery
York Hospital
16 Hospital Drive, Suite A
York, ME 03909, USA

E-mail address:
rmartin@yorkhospital.com

costs, disparities and specialties beyond colorectal surgery. Simply put, enhanced recovery provides not just high-quality care, but high-value care.

The future of enhanced recovery is bright. Even since these chapters were written, new advances have been made in fields including cardiac surgery, neonatology and thoracic surgery. Key organizations such as the ERAS® Society and American Society of Enhanced Recovery (ASER) continue to champion and push the frontier. Technology is also coming to the forefront and being leveraged to ensure even better implementation and auditing of recovery processes. The next generation of healthcare providers, from surgeons and anesthesiologists to nurses and allied health professionals, will have a solid foundation to build even more effective recovery programs.

I would like to thank the many authors for their important contributions and look forward to seeing the many good things to come as we strive to recover our surgical patients and families in the best way.

Sincerely,

Daniel I. Chu, MD, FACS, FASCRS
Division of Gastrointestinal Surgery
Department of Surgery
University of Alabama at Birmingham
KB427
1720 2nd Avenue South
Birmingham, AL 35294, USA

E-mail address:
dchu@uab.edu

Overview of Enhanced Recovery After Surgery

The Evolution and Adoption of Enhanced Recovery After Surgery in North America

Julie Thacker, MD

KEYWORDS

- ERAS • Enhanced Recovery After Surgery • Perioperative medicine
- Best surgical outcomes • United States • Health care costs • Enhanced Recovery

KEY POINTS

- Enhanced Recovery is broadly defined as the application of evidence based perioperative care elements for improved surgical outcomes.
- Demonstration of perioperative physiology and modifiable surgical stress with innovation of surgical technique, in combination with pressure to drive down health care costs, have coalesced into a unique version of perioperative medicine in the United States.
- The US government has failed to show interest; there are no performance metrics, no participation requirements, and certainly no monetary incentives for implementation of best perioperative practices.
- When considering the term, Enhanced Recovery is, in its broadest sense, an amalgam of industry, innovation, patient-focused care, cost-effective strategies, and collaboration with a goal of best perioperative outcomes.

Ever striving to perform the best operation and to provide the best perioperative care is inherent to the surgeon personality. Why did we adopt principles of handwashing, antisepsis, and then aseptic technique? Why do we debate the effectiveness of surgical headdress? Why do we benchmark, compare, and compete to prove best care? Why do we prepare the colon for a colon resection or challenge immediate postoperative enteral diets?[1–4]

The answer to any of these questions is, again, found in the surgeon's drive for best care. Over the past 2.5 decades, this drive has been variably defined by perioperative quality, value care in surgery, and outcome effectiveness. The coined phrase, Enhanced Recovery, has been applied to the application of perioperative care principles for best surgical outcomes.[5]

The author has nothing to disclose.
Duke University Health Center, Department of Surgery, DUMC, HAFS 7678, Durham, NC 27710, USA
E-mail address: julie.thacker@duke.edu

Surg Clin N Am 98 (2018) 1109–1117
https://doi.org/10.1016/j.suc.2018.07.016
0039-6109/18/© 2018 Elsevier Inc. All rights reserved.

surgical.theclinics.com

DEFINITIONS AND HISTORY

Defined as continuous improvement in perioperative care, Enhanced Recovery has served as a term to reference efforts in the perioperative space. A discussion of the adoption of Enhanced Recovery in the United States could broadly course through the history of surgery. For purposes herein, Enhanced Recovery is limited to the work referencing the actual term, and, for completeness, we start with definitions, history, and the aspects of surgical care in the United States that created the context for adoption of Enhanced Recovery unique to our medical system.

Enhanced Recovery in the United States is distinct to, yet interwoven with, the use of the term internationally. Dependent on context, the definition of Enhanced Recovery is best described as the application of perioperative care principles to the continuum of surgical care with the goal of best surgical outcomes. While US surgeon scientists explored surgical stress and response to trauma, US anesthesiologist-scientists experimented with blood management theories and intraoperative fluid strategies. Efforts in Europe were on parallel, and often collaborative tracks. Specifically, many tenets of Enhanced Recovery are based on the work of Boston surgeon, Doug Wilmore, and Danish surgeon, Henrik Kehlet. Copublishing on the physiologic response to surgical stress, they pondered the potential benefits of managing, reacting to, or even actively reducing this stress. In so doing, they proposed that recovering from surgery could be less physiologically complicated, or, in other words, enhanced.[6–11]

Applying the principle of decreasing surgical stress to his personal colorectal surgery practice, Kehlet and Mogensen[12] published astounding results of a 23-hour hospital stay after colectomy, in 1999. With a very intentional, surgeon-driven approach to minimizing insulin resistance and minimizing starvation, in combination with optimizing activity, Kehlet and Mogensen[12] showed decreased time to return of bowel function after colectomy. This one perioperative perimeter, time to return of bowel function, has since been shown to be the main driver of length of stay after colectomy. Kehlet then associated decreased length of stay with improvements in an array of surgical outcomes of interest, including surgical and medical complications. Initially, denied publication in traditional surgical journals, Kehlet[13] published in the *British Journal of Anesthesia*, largely avoiding attention by the US surgical academic audience.

"Enhanced Recovery After Surgery"

His work was noticed, however, by his Scandinavian neighbors, who shared his history of studying surgical stress response and metabolism. In early 2000s, the ERAS (Enhanced Recovery After Surgery) Study Group was formed to attempt adoption of Professor Kehlet's work at their home institutions, including Karolinska and Tromso.[14] Although not initially successful in replicating Kehlet's outcomes, this effort significantly and transparently reported the need for local adaptations, inclusion care paradigms, and continuous auditing. Over the following decade, the ERAS Working Group and Research Group, became the ERAS® Society with a focus on defining generalizable principles of perioperative care with a focus of decreasing surgical stress and improving outcomes.[15–17] Publications of their experience and their guidelines (2010–2013), catapulted the term, "ERAS," to general use. Enhanced Recovery After Surgery and ERAS are trademarked terms owned by the ERAS® Society; however, these are readily used in perioperative literature when referring to the principles of this work.[18–22]

Evidence-Based Perioperative Medicine

Predating the ERAS® Society, evidence-based perioperative medicine (EBPOM) defines the anesthesia aspect of perioperative care in the United Kingdom, producing meetings and educational conferences to forward the science and implementation of perioperative medicine. Since 1997, EBPOM, a not-for-profit collaborative project between a number of UK and international academic institutions, has promoted the examination, discussion, and application of evidence-based medicine to perioperative care (EBPOM.org). Their goal is leading skills acquisition and adoption of best practices, and their work has included the anesthesia components of Enhanced Recovery with a broader perioperative medicine scope. More recently, in close collaboration with ASER, the American Society for Enhanced Recovery, EBPOM-ASER have more fully addressed the perioperative medicine continuum, with specific attention to surgical outcomes via a broader viewing lens.

ENHANCED RECOVERY IN THE UNITED STATES

On the aforementioned US work in metabolism, surgical stress, and intraoperative fluid,[23,24] we had 2 related forces driving change in our country's perioperative care paradigm. Quality outcomes and technologic innovation weave integral foundation to much of US surgical improvement efforts, and Enhanced Recovery has been no exception. Related to the technologic advances in the operating room, technology related to patient care processes, auditing, and imposed improvement strategies are also important to implementation timing and success.[25–28]

Impact of Laparoscopy on Enhanced Recovery Adoption in the United States

Beginning with adoption of laparoscopic techniques for gynecologic and straightforward biliary procedures, physically minimizing the stress of abdominopelvic surgery has been a focus of US surgical innovation since the mid-1980s. Steep adoption curve for laparoscopic cholecystectomy and appendectomy, mirrored even in training programs, opened the minds of US surgeons to expect different recovery patterns. Patients required drastically less analgesia. Equally impressive reductions in hospital length of stay were realized. As most of abdominopelvic operations in the United States are performed by busy, nonacademic, general surgeons and gynecologists, the time-saving application of common care principles spread. If a patient undergoing a laparoscopic cholecystectomy can eat on postoperative day 1, can a laparoscopic colectomy patient eat on postoperative day 1 as well? A very organic spread of concept occurred during the postoperative phase of patients cared for by laparoscopic surgeons, including those reporting 23-hour colectomies, just like Henrik Kehlet.[29] The American difference, however, was that we defined the etiology of better outcomes as surgical approach, not perioperative care. Throughout the 1990s and early 2000s, advanced laparoscopic surgeons reported decreased need for analgesia, decreased length of stay, decreased wound complications, and, to counter nay-sayers, they eventually declared decreased costs for laparoscopic approaches to traditionally open operations. These reports credit the decreased surgical stress of technique with the patient's subsequent tolerance and self-defined postoperative course of early diet and ambulation.[20–22]

In Europe, the principle of encouraging patients undergoing traditional approach operations (open laparotomy) to eat and move early after operation, was coined Enhanced Recovery After Surgery. The evolving US practice of allowing post-laparoscopic procedure patients to eat and move was resulting in similar outcome without a tagged dictum or care campaign.

Impact of Costs and System Influences

The most notable difference in the adoption of Enhanced Recovery, between Europe and the United States, is rooted in the second driver of care paradigm change.

Although the differences in payer system and the amount of gross national product spent on health care between the United States and any other country in the world can explain many developments and deficiencies in our system, it was actually in similarity that the efforts of the United Kingdom and United States became aligned with regard to "ERAS." As described by the National Health Service (NHS) lead anesthetist, Monty Mythen, UK reached a health care budget crisis.[30] This crisis forced the nation's health care system into minimal spending mode; Mythen, and his surgeon counterpart, Alan Horgan, were charged with decreasing perioperative costs. A starting focus was length of stay. More complicated, yet also more important, they focused overall efforts on decreasing complications. Over the course of 2009 to 2011, the Enhanced Recovery Partnership Programme encouraged the adoption of basic Enhanced Recovery principles across most surgical units in the NHS in England. With this, implementation strategies and successes were broadcast, and cost savings were recognized and reported. Success of coordinated, evidence-based care to decrease surgical stress was declared standard of care. Lack of implementation of Enhanced Recovery principles of care became substandard in the NHS. Sustaining strategies, quality audits, and improvement programs persist in the UK environment of intentional bundling of best evidence-based perioperative practices.[31]

Although the impact of perioperative pain on recovery was recognized by the ERAS Working Group reports and the US-based laparoscopists, neither surgeon-led effort was well connected to the specialists of analgesia; that is, until the UK multidisciplinary team built their model. The basis of the work in the United Kingdom was cost savings by complication minimization. The focus was not on scientific discovery or reporting, nor on innovation. The relationship between surgical and anesthesia team, with the continued engagement and guidance of nursing as modeled in the 1990s in Denmark, describes the current wave of US Enhanced Recovery endeavor. The recognition that every action of every team member of the surgical journey impacts outcomes has been daunting and guiding. From the growth of innovation partnered with science at academic institutions to health care management strategies of for-profit systems, Enhanced Recovery has become US jargon for doing everything around surgery better. Better than what? This is not well defined. Better than who? At least better than competitors or academic rivals. Better for whom, though? Regardless of the publication site, author source, or population of interest, Enhanced Recovery continues to prove the better way to provide perioperative care.

American College of Surgeons, American College of Surgeons National Quality Improvement Program, American Society of Anesthesiologists–Perioperative Surgical Home, Society of American Gastrointestinal and Endoscopic Surgeons, and Impact of Medical Societies

The Society of American Gastrointestinal and Endoscopic Surgeons (SAGES) recently reported that 30% of surveyed US surgeons responded that they did not recognize the term, Enhanced Recovery (SAGES SMART, www.sages.org/smart-enhanced-recovery-program/). Obviously, spread of Enhanced Recovery, at least by name, is not considered ubiquitous. However, US hospital reports regarding implementation of Enhanced Recovery has exploded over the past decade. As reported at the American College of Surgeons National Quality Improvement Program (NSQIP) Conference, publications on Enhanced Recovery from US-based authors skyrocketed in number and in percentage of all worldwide publications. More similar still to the UK work, 2009 to 2012, US publications focused on length of stay and costs and usually referred to a multidisciplinary team. Out of the focus on laparoscopy and distinct from the surgeon-led Scandinavian hospitals, teams with at least a surgeon, anesthesiologist, lead nurse or coordinator, and an administrator were considered crucial to the work. Exceptions to this approach have faltered. The American Society of Anesthesiologists created the "PSH, Perioperative Surgical Home," in response to threatening payment schemes that dosed payments relative to recognized work effort. The PSH, in an attempt to identify all possible revenue streams for anesthesiologists, claimed to have the patient-focused perioperative care principles. With a strong base in managing orthopedic patient perioperative medical issues during preoperative and postoperative care, the perioperative surgical home failed to capture most abdominopelvic operations performed by surgeons who self-managed their patients from diagnosis to return to baseline. This failure to collaborate plagued the PSH effort, despite many great PSH ideas regarding preoperative optimization for orthopedic surgical candidates. Similarly, individual institutions document their struggles with lack of service engagement. In the United States, a unique challenge to change management is motivation to collaborate. Fee-for-service structure does not encourage shared effort across billable service lines. If a recommendation costs money or time, significant challenges exist to harness ownership and maintenance. At the core, we all want to do what is best for the patient; however, our system wants to get paid for this effort. If anesthesia effort, surgery effort, and nursing effort are each unequally represented by remuneration, it is very difficult to motivate each team to participate equally. Also challenging is that Enhanced Recovery implementation and, even more so, sustainability, takes specialty-specific motivation. Anesthesiologists need to motivate and to help define the anesthesia care components in an Enhanced Recovery protocol. Surgeons need to motivate surgeons, and nurses are essential to drive pathways, education, and nursing outreach.[25]

As an attempt to create an Enhanced Recovery "toolbox," the American College of Surgeons' NSQIP proposed an Enhanced Recovery in NSQIP, "ERIN," program to study implementation of Enhanced Recovery principles in colon surgery at NSQIP hospitals. Although results showed expected improvements at the participating centers, an interesting detail behind the study was the centers that did not participate. In the initial creation of the program, 46 programs expressed interest. The study start-up meeting required a representative from each of the disciplines to be involved in the creation of the Enhanced Recovery program at the center: nursing, anesthesia, surgery, and administration. We dropped to 24 sites before the start-up meeting; we dropped to 19 sites before going live. In this free-to-participants, Enhanced Recovery coaching and implementation offer, via a service already in place at the hospitals approached, more than half of the interested teams dropped out because they were not able to secure participation from each specialty. Deeper review revealed that the lack of support was either surgery or anesthesia; nursing and administration were uniformly willing to attend sessions and support effort necessary for the project.[26]

SHARED CHALLENGES AT THE NATIONAL LEVEL

Difficulty of management and adequate specialty representation are realized at the national level of multidisciplinary societies as well. Surgical specialty societies rarely invite anesthesia or nursing presenters to their podiums. Anesthesia societies rely on anesthesiologists to present work on preoperative optimization, whereas most of this work occurs via the surgery clinic, before a traditional anesthesia team meets a surgical candidate. Likewise, the nursing societies present perioperative topics of nursing interest without surgeons or anesthesiologist or patient outcome research playing much of a role.

AMERICAN SOCIETY FOR ENHANCED RECOVERY: LEARNING TO COLLABORATE

An interest in multidisciplinary promotion of best perioperative outcomes has been led by ASER, the American Society for Enhanced Recovery (www.enhancedrecovery. org). With a mandatorily diverse board and alternating president status of specialty, ASER attempts to study and present patient-focused perioperative care. Having a particular interest in promoting the science from which guidelines and protocols are created, ASER interacts with surgical, anesthesia, certified registered nurse anesthetist (CRNA), and nursing societies to forcibly intermingle our influences for best outcomes. Established in 2014, ASER represents the society version of adoption of Enhanced Recovery in the United States and hopes to promote best practices via collaboration.

A notable academic effort that arose from the leaders of ASER and EBPOM is POQI, the PeriOperative Quality Initiative (www.POQI.org). The premise of POQI is derived from ADQI, the Acute Dialysis Quality Initiative. The model is a modified Delphi method for expert opinion on important topics on daily patient care for the surgical patient. Each of the 16 manuscripts (10 published, 6 in peer review), has nursing, CRNA, surgery, and anesthesia authors. Particularly aware of US health care strategies, the investigators have written with understanding of cost structures in the United States, interactions of siloed stakeholders, and shared outcomes without shared inflow of resources. This commitment to multidisciplinary representation of specialty for best perioperative guidelines is unique and impactful.

INTERNATIONAL INTEREST IN THE US ADOPTION OF ENHANCED RECOVERY

As detailed previously, the growth of Enhanced Recovery as a named perioperative quality improvement focus in the United States in many ways mimicked the 2009 to 2011 UK Partnership Programme. Notably, the US attempt has been without national drive or data, however. Without government-imposed collaboration, our efforts have grown within our existing financial siloes. Through academic and third-party payer support, though, collaborative efforts are increasing. Parallel to the maturation of the relationship between ASER and EBPOM, EBPOM-US has initiated masters training courses across the United States this year. The ERAS® Society also has a US chapter that began in 2017. Juxtaposed to the American-based, intentionally specialty mixed, ASER, and the anesthesia-strong, EBPOM, ERAS-US is surgeon project, with a strong presence of their European base.

CURRENT DIRECTIONS

The analogy of Enhanced Recovery implementation to the uptake of laparoscopy can be extended to include the impact of industry support, third-party payer involvement, and patient-driven outreach. However, noticeably, the US government has failed to show interest. There are no performance metrics, no participation requirements, and certainly no monetary reward or incentive for implementation of Enhanced Recovery. Small academic grants and society support have led studies. Exceptionally, an impressive US Agency for Healthcare Research and Quality grant was awarded (2017–2020) to a team of Enhanced Recovery experts. The goal of the work is implementation guidance across hundreds of US hospitals. Hopefully, more such funding will be realized to continue the development of perioperative medicine and implementation science in the United States.

In addition to the lack of research support, the lack of or incentivized implementation requirement from the US government makes a national, unified Enhanced Recovery program unlikely in the United States. Eventual adoption of Enhanced Recovery principles as our new routine care is insidious, however, via substantive, unfunded academic effort. Inculcation of new generations of providers is occurring with incorporation of Enhanced Recovery principles into training programs and even certification programs for surgeons, anesthesiologists, nurse anesthetists, and nurses. Examples include continuing education programs and the colorectal surgery certification examinations have included Enhanced Recovery topics for the past 5 years. New to the United States, anesthesia fellowships in perioperative medicine also drive this education. Unlike the government administration of US trauma systems or the industry and surgeon-led development of laparoscopy, the adoption of Enhanced Recovery is most strongly driven by quality comparators and individual provider/individual health care system effort. Yet, with reinforcement via our certification process, incorporation of principles into practice is growing and will be sustainable.

Demonstration of perioperative physiology and modifiable surgical stress with innovation of surgical technique and the pressure to drive down health care costs have coalesced to a unique version of perioperative medicine in the United States. When considering the term, Enhanced Recovery, is, in its broadest sense, an amalgam of industry, innovation, patient-focused caring, cost-effective strategies, and collaboration with a goal of best perioperative outcomes. The adoption of Enhanced Recovery may have truly started with adoption of handwashing, while it is our hope that it is soon recognized as "business as usual."

REFERENCES

1. Statement on Operating Room Attire, ACS position statement. 2016. Available at: www.facs.org/about-acs/statements/87-surgical-attire. Accessed August 4, 2016.
2. Klinger AL, Green H, Monlezun DJ, et al. The role of bowel preparation in colorectal surgery: results of the 2012-2015 ACS-NSQIP data. Ann Surg 2017. https://doi.org/10.1097/SLA.0000000000002568.
3. Evidence-based Practice Center Systematic Review Protocol. Project Title: Oral Mechanical Bowel Preparation for Colorectal Surgery. Available at: http://effectivehealthcare.ahrq.gov. Accessed March 26, 2013.
4. Fujii T, Morita H, Sutoh T, et al. Benefit of oral feeding as early as one day after elective surgery for colorectal cancer: oral feeding on first versus second postoperative day. Int Surg 2014;99(3):211–5.
5. Lemanu DP, Singh PP, Stowers MD, et al. A systematic review to assess cost effectiveness of enhanced recovery after surgery programmes in colorectal surgery. Colorectal Dis 2014;16(5):338–46.
6. Basse L, Hjort Jakobsen D, Billesbølle P, et al. A clinical pathway to accelerate recovery after colonic resection. Ann Surg 2000;232(1):51–7.
7. Kehlet H, Wilmore DW. Evidence-based surgical care and the evolution of fast-track surgery. Ann Surg 2008;248(2):189–98.
8. Wilmore DW. Today in surgical practice: a conversation with Prof. Henrik Kehlet. Bull Am Coll Surg 2001;86(8):27–8, 31.
9. Kehlet H, Wilmore DW. Fast-track surgery. Br J Surg 2005;92(1):3–4.
10. Kehlet H, Wilmore DW. Multimodal strategies to improve surgical outcome. Am J Surg 2002;183(6):630–41.
11. Wilmore DW, Kehlet H. Management of patients in fast track surgery. BMJ 2001; 322(7284):473–6.

12. Kehlet H, Mogensen T. Hospital stay of 2 days after open sigmoidectomy with a multimodal rehabilitation programme. Br J Surg 1999;86(2):227–30.
13. Kehlet H. Surgical stress: the role of pain and analgesia. Br J Anaesth 1989;63(2): 189–95.
14. Ljungqvist O, Young-Fadok T, Demartines N. The history of enhanced recovery after surgery and the ERAS society. J Laparoendosc Adv Surg Tech A 2017; 27(9):860–2.
15. Lassen K, Hannemann P, Ljungqvist O, Enhanced Recovery After Surgery Group. Patterns in current perioperative practice: survey of colorectal surgeons in five northern European countries. BMJ 2005;330(7505):1420–1.
16. Fearon KC, Ljungqvist O, Von Meyenfeldt M, et al. Enhanced recovery after surgery: a consensus review of clinical care for patients undergoing colonic resection. Clin Nutr 2005;24(3):466–77.
17. Nygren J, Hausel J, Kehlet H, et al. A comparison in five European centres of case mix, clinical management and outcomes following either conventional or fast-track perioperative care in colorectal surgery. Clin Nutr 2005;24(3):455–61.
18. Varadhan KK, Lobo DN, Ljungqvist O. Enhanced recovery after surgery: the future of improving surgical care. Crit Care Clin 2010;26(3):527–47.
19. Gustafsson UO, Scott MJ, Schwenk W, Enhanced Recovery After Surgery Society. Guidelines for perioperative care in elective colonic surgery: Enhanced Recovery After Surgery (ERAS®) Society recommendations. Clin Nutr 2012;31(6): 783–800.
20. Nygren J, Thacker J, Carli F, et al, Enhanced Recovery After Surgery (ERAS) Society, for Perioperative Care; European Society for Clinical Nutrition and Metabolism (ESPEN); International Association for Surgical Metabolism and Nutrition (IASMEN). Guidelines for perioperative care in elective rectal/pelvic surgery: Enhanced recovery after surgery (ERAS(®)) Society recommendations. World J Surg 2013;37(2):285–305.
21. Gustafsson UO, Scott MJ, Schwenk W, et al, Enhanced Recovery After Surgery (ERAS) Society, for Perioperative Care; European Society for Clinical Nutrition and Metabolism (ESPEN); International Association for Surgical Metabolism and Nutrition (IASMEN). Guidelines for perioperative care in elective colonic surgery: Enhanced Recovery After Surgery (ERAS(®)) Society recommendations. World J Surg 2013;37(2):259–84.
22. Lassen K, Coolsen MM, Slim K, et al, Enhanced Recovery After Surgery (ERAS) Society, for Perioperative Care; European Society for Clinical Nutrition and Metabolism (ESPEN); International Association for Surgical Metabolism and Nutrition (IASMEN). Guidelines for perioperative care for pancreaticoduodenectomy: Enhanced Recovery After Surgery (ERAS®) Society recommendations. World J Surg 2013;37(2):240–58.
23. Roche AM, Miller TE, Gan TJ. Goal-directed fluid management with transoesophageal Doppler. Best Pract Res Clin Anaesthesiol 2009;23(3):327–34.
24. Moretti EW, Robertson KM, El-Moalem H, et al. Intraoperative colloid administration reduces postoperative nausea and vomiting and improves postoperative outcomes compared with crystalloid administration. Anesth Analg 2003;96(2):611–7.
25. London MJ, Shroyer AL, Jernigan V, et al. Fast-track cardiac surgery in a Department of Veterans Affairs patient population. Ann Thorac Surg 1997;64(1):134–41.
26. Kehlet H, Büchler MW, Beart RW Jr, et al. Care after colonic operation—is it evidence-based? Results from a multinational survey in Europe and the United States. J Am Coll Surg 2006;202(1):45–54.

27. Kariv Y, Delaney CP, Senagore AJ, et al. Clinical outcomes and cost analysis of a "fast track" postoperative care pathway for ileal pouch-anal anastomosis: a case control study. Dis Colon Rectum 2007;50(2):137–46.
28. Bosio RM, Smith BM, Aybar PS, et al. Implementation of laparoscopic colectomy with fast-track care in an academic medical center: benefits of a fully ascended learning curve and specialty expertise. Am J Surg 2007;193(3):413–5 [discussion: 415–6].
29. Augestad KM, Delaney CP. Postoperative ileus: impact of pharmacological treatment, laparoscopic surgery and enhanced recovery pathways. World J Gastroenterol 2010;16(17):2067–74.
30. Mythen MG. Enhanced Recovery in the NHS. Presented at the ASER World Congress. Washington DC, April 24, 2014.
31. Simpson JC, Moonesinghe SR, Grocott MP, National Enhanced Recovery Partnership Advisory Board. Enhanced recovery from surgery in the UK: an audit of the enhanced recovery partnership programme 2009-2012. Br J Anaesth 2015;115(4):560–8.

Enhanced Recovery After Surgery and Effects on Quality Metrics

Jessica Y. Liu, MD, MS[a,b],*, Elizabeth C. Wick, MD[c]

KEYWORDS

- Enhanced recovery after surgery • Quality metrics • Adherence
- Hospital-acquired infections • Patient-reported outcomes • Readmission

KEY POINTS

- Enhanced recovery after surgery (ERAS) bundles decrease physiologic stress response to surgery and maintain postoperative physiologic function.
- ERAS improves surgical quality by impacting quality metrics such as length of stay, hospital-acquired infections, readmissions, and patient experience.
- ERAS is a bundle, and better adherence leads to improvement in quality metrics.
- Auditing and interdisciplinary collaboration are important components of successful ERAS implementation.

INTRODUCTION

As health care evolves and improves care delivery to patients, poor surgical outcomes are no longer considered just an inevitable occurrence after surgery. The quality of health care is now assessed utilizing quality metrics, and these quality metrics are also used to compare the quality of different health care organizations.[1] Quality metrics also now play a large role in health care and reimbursements in health care, with physicians being incentivized to improve their care through pay-for-performance incentive programs.[2] Although quality metrics can refer to a broad range of definitions, one of the most popular models of quality metrics was described by Donabedian in 1966 and is now known as the Donabedian model. Donabedian described quality assessment by describing 3 categories of quality metrics: structure, process, and outcomes.[3] Structural measures

Disclosure Statement: Jessica Y. Liu and Elizabeth C. Wick receive salary support through a contract with Agency for Healthcare Research & Quality (HHSP233201500020I).

[a] American College of Surgeons, Division of Research and Optimal Patient Care, 633 North St Clair Street, 22nd Floor, Chicago, IL 60611, USA; [b] Department of Surgery, Emory University, 1364 Clifton Road NE, Room H127, Atlanta, GA 30322, USA; [c] Division of General Surgery, University of California San Francisco, 513 Parnassus Avenue, Room HSW1601, San Francisco, CA 94143, USA
* Corresponding author. American College of Surgeons, 633 North St Clair Street, 22nd Floor, Chicago, IL 60611.
E-mail address: jessica.liu@facs.org

Surg Clin N Am 98 (2018) 1119–1127
https://doi.org/10.1016/j.suc.2018.07.001
0039-6109/18/© 2018 Elsevier Inc. All rights reserved.

refer to the material and human resources and organizational structure required to provide health care; process measures refer to the actions that are performed in order to provide or receive health-care, and outcome measures refer to the effect health care has on the health status of those who are receiving health care.[3] Applying enhanced recovery after surgery (ERAS) to the Donabedian model, the evidence-based individual elements of ERAS® protocols are process measures that aim to decrease the physiologic stress response to surgery and maintain postoperative physiologic function, thereby improving outcome measures and improving surgical quality.

PATHOPHYSIOLOGY

The effect of ERAS on quality metrics is well studied and has been shown to lead to significant improvement. Several systematic reviews have been performed comparing ERAS with traditional perioperative care in mortality, morbidity, length of stay (LOS), and readmission rates.[4–6] Although there was no statistically significant improvement found in mortality, a decrease in postoperative morbidity of 48% (relative risk [RR] 0.52, 95% confidence interval [CI] 0.38–0.71)[6] and 47% (RR 0.53, 95% CI 0.41–0.69)[7] was found. Additionally, LOS was decreased by −2.94 days (−3.92 to −2.19)[6] and −2.51 days (−3.54 to −1.47).[7] This decrease in morbidity and LOS was not associated with any increase in hospital readmissions (3.3%–4.4% vs 4.2%–5.7%).[6,7]

The Pathophysiology of Enhanced Recovery After Surgery

These improvements in outcomes can be attributed to the pathophysiology of ERAS. One of the known effects of surgery is postoperative immunosuppression in addition to a physiologic stress response the body has to surgery.[8,9] After the tissue injury associated with surgery, the systemic inflammatory response is activated and leads to a proinflammatory state.[10] ERAS has been shown to have a statistically significant reduction in inflammatory markers interleukin (IL)-6 and C-reactive protein (CRP), and also demonstrated that compared with conventional patients, they may have improved humoral and cellular immunity.[2] The various elements of ERAS were designed to prevent stress, reduce the surgical stress response, preserve physiologic function, and promote a quick return to baseline.[11] These actions combined lead to decreased complications and improved outcomes.

Decreasing Hyperglycemia and Insulin Resistance

One of the results of the surgical stress response is its impact on postoperative insulin resistance and hyperglycemia. Increased insulin resistance and hyperglycemia have been found to be associated with complications and increased LOS.[12] The use of preoperative carbohydrate loading and reduction of overnight fasting demonstrated that insulin sensitivity would increase and lead to less insulin resistance in the postoperative period.[13] Additionally, other ERAS components like reducing postoperative nausea and vomiting (PONV) with antiemetic prophylaxis to improve oral intake of nutrients, reducing ileus rates and the stress response by decreasing opioid use with regional blocks and epidurals, and adequate fluid status maintenance to support bowel function all contribute to decreased hyperglycemia.[14] A Cochrane review found an association between hospital LOS and preoperative carbohydrate loading, with a reduced LOS of 1 to 1.5 days.[15]

LENGTH OF STAY

One of the quality metrics that ERAS has demonstrated the most significant impact on is overall hospital LOS. The use of an ERAS bundle has been demonstrated to significantly reduce LOS in patients.[16] The ERAS elements that contribute to decreased LOS are multifactorial and spread over all the phases of care. Preoperatively, the use of preadmission counseling and education serves to inform patients and their families on the expectations following surgery and the milestones they would be encouraged to meet, thereby helping them meet the criteria for discharge sooner.[14] Intraoperatively, goal-directed fluid resuscitation and reduction of nasogastric tube (NGT) use all act toward reducing LOS. Postoperatively, a focus on preventing PONV and reduced fasting all impact the LOS positively. It is also probable that reduction in opioid use and increased use of multimodal analgesia contribute to the improvements seen in this metric, because many of the other ERAS processes hinge on optimal pain management and reduced opioid use. This decreased LOS with ERAS has been demonstrated in not just colorectal patients, but across various different surgeries.[16]

Postoperative Nausea and Vomiting

One of the major causes of delayed discharge from the hospital is PONV, with an incidence rate as high as 70% in postoperative patients in some studies.[17] The use of antiemetic prophylaxis and other anesthesia techniques to minimize PONV in ERAS therefore has a positive impact on LOS.[18] There is an association between opioid use and PONV, so ERAS components such as using epidurals and reducing opioid use with multimodal analgesia also serve to decrease PONV and reduce LOS. Additionally, minimizing preoperative fasting, having preoperative carbohydrate loading, and maintaining adequate hydration in patients all contribute to decreasing PONV.[19]

Reduction of Ileus

Another common cause that leads to increased LOS by delaying discharge is postoperative ileus. In a Cochrane review, epidural local anesthetic was shown to have a decreased time to return of gastrointestinal function compared with opioid-based regimens by an average of 17.5 hours with better pain control.[20] Another meta-analysis found that epidural use reduced ileus by an average of 36 hours.[21] Another ERAS element that has been shown to reduce ileus is goal-directed fluid management, both intraoperatively and postoperatively. A more restrictive fluid management in patients has been shown to decrease ileus, with return of flatus occurring on average 1 day faster and stool an average of 2 days faster.[22,23] The average hospitalization length was 3 days longer in those who did not have restrictive fluid management.[23] Eliminating the routine placement of NGTs[24] in ERAS is significantly associated with earlier return of bowel function and aligns well with reducing fasting in postoperative patients.[25,26]

HOSPITAL-ACQUIRED INFECTION

ERAS has been shown to impact rates of preventable harms like hospital-acquired infections (HAIs). The annual cost is estimated at $9.8 billion for HAIs, and so reducing HAIs not only decreases patient morbidity but can have financial benefit to the hospital, and is a component of many value-based purchasing programs and is also one of the main focuses of public reporting.[2] The presence of 1 HAI, such as a surgical site infection (SSI), can make a patient more prone to another HAI, such as catheter-associated urinary tract infection (CAUTI), and tends to cascade and cluster, so reducing HAI through ERAS also reduces the snowball effect of acquiring an HAI to begin with.[2]

Surgical Site Infections

In a meta-analysis evaluating the effect of ERAS compared with traditional care, ERAS was found to significantly reduce the rates of SSI (RR 0.75, 95% CI 0.58–0.98, P=.04).[2] ERAS® recommendations include the use of preincision intravenous antibiotics, as well as skin preparation,[14] which has been shown to drastically improve SSI rates following surgery.[27] A Cochrane review evaluating prophylactic antibiotic use in colorectal surgery patients found high-quality evidence that prophylactic antibiotic use decreased SSI rates by as much as 75%.[28] Additionally, hypothermia has been found to be associated with higher rates of wound infection, and so maintaining normothermia, another component of ERAS, is an important contributor to reducing SSI rates. The reduction of fasting in ERAS and avoiding a malnourished state has also been shown to decrease inflammation and physiologic stress, and has been associated with improved wound healing and decreased rates of SSI as well.[4,29] Additionally, most of the recent SSI prevention guidelines published have included a bundled approach to prevention as an intervention. ERAS programs provide great opportunity to layer SSI prevention bundles into pathways and promote standardization and compliance.

Pneumonia

A significant reduction in pneumonia was found when comparing ERAS with conventional perioperative care in a systematic review and meta-analysis (RR 0.38, 95% CI 0.23–0.61, P<.001).[2] Epidural use has been found to be protective against the development of pneumonia by improving blood oxygenation and lung function.[30] Additionally, the use of epidurals minimizes the need for opioids, which has been shown to decrease the rate of pulmonary complications and pneumonia.[31,32] Reducing opioid use also contributes to early mobilization, another component of ERAS, and has been shown to be associated with decreased rates of chest complications.[33]

Urinary Tract Infection

The early removal of urinary bladder catheters has been found on multiple meta-analyses to reduce rates of CAUTI.[34] In particular, the use of a reminder or stop order was found to be effective at reducing prolonged urinary bladder catheterization.[35] The successful implementation of ERAS involves integrating interventions such as a reminder or stop order for bladder catheterization into a provider's daily work flow. Undergoing surgery in general remains an opportunistic scenario for the development of urinary tract infection (UTI). Preincision antibiotics have been found to be associated with reduced UTI rates, and the reduction of other HAIs such as SSI also leads to a reduction in UTIs that can result secondary to other HAIs.[2]

READMISSIONS

Unplanned readmission following surgery is thought to likely be a result of early postoperative complications related to the surgery.[36] Readmissions are also tracked as a part of most value-based purchasing programs, and reducing unplanned readmission rates is gaining prioritization as a quality metric to target for improvement. A common misperception about ERAS is that it reduces LOS while increasing hospital readmission rates. In a meta-analysis comparing ERAS patients with those receiving conventional postoperative care, there was a significant decrease in LOS while maintaining similar readmission rates between the 2 groups.[4] Although readmission rates remained the same, 1 observational study evaluated the reasons for readmission following ERAS and demonstrated that with the decreased rates of postoperative SSI in ERAS there was a subsequent reduction in postoperative readmissions for SSI as well (7.3% vs 16.6%, $P=.01$).[16] When evaluating predictors of readmission, preoperative chemoradiotherapy and decreased adherence to ERAS components were found to be associated with unplanned readmissions.[37] The most common cause for readmission was postoperative ileus.[16,37] Interestingly, in those who were readmitted in a study by Fabrizio and colleagues,[16] the total LOS between the initial hospitalization and the readmission was comparable to the average LOS in those who were not participating in ERAS at all, indicating that the beneficial effects of ERAS on LOS comprised what was lost in those who were readmitted without increasing total hospital days.

Additionally, utilizing preoperative patient education and counseling to discuss patients' anticipated discharge needs allow for more time to ensure a coordinated discharge plan, with a patient having all the assistance he or she needs to successfully recover and avoid readmission. A study by Fredericks and Yau[38] showed that individualized patient education compared with a standardized patient education packet was associated with decreased readmission rates in cardiac patients. In addition to patient-specific education, procedure-specific education is also another targeted education strategy that has shown improvements in readmission rates. Patients receiving new ileostomies at Beth Israel Deaconess Medical Center were targeted with ileostomy-specific education, and this was shown to significantly decrease readmissions, especially readmissions for dehydration.[39]

PATIENT EXPERIENCE

One quality metric that is currently gaining momentum is the measurement of patient experience through surveys such as the Hospital Consumer Assessment of Healthcare Providers and Systems (HCAHPS). Patient experience is a significant component of the US Centers for Medicare and Medicaid Services (CMS) Star Rating on Patient Safety metric. Despite a decreased LOS, the use of ERAS has not been found to impact patients' perceptions of discharge readiness or transition of care negatively.[16] One key component that likely contributes to improved patient experience is the focus of ERAS on patient education and preadmission counseling. By educating patients and their families prior to surgery on expected in-hospital milestones and expectations upon discharge to home, and then reinforcing these concepts throughout hospitalization, patients are more likely to feel comfortable with their hospital experience and their transitions of care. Furthermore, there is emerging evidence that patients tend to perceive their care in a more positive frame if they felt that their care was coordinated, and their providers exhibited strong teamwork. Transdisciplinary ERAS implementation teams are some of the best examples of teamwork in surgery. Furthermore, standardization and reduction in variation of care help all team members align and message similarly, and this is received positively by patients.

In fact, some studies suggest that patient experience is actually positively impacted by participating in ERAS. In one study from the University of Virginia using Press Ganey surveys, Thiele and colleagues[40] found that after ERAS implementation, their overall survey scores increased from the 29th percentile to the 59th percentile. More patients reported feeling ready for discharge (increasing from 41st percentile to 99th percentile), and satisfaction with pain control increased (43rd to 98th percentile); additionally, patients reported a higher likelihood of recommending that hospital to others (32nd to 89th percentile).[40] Patients' perception of their nurse's response to their pain was also positively impacted despite a focus of ERAS on decreased opioid use, with patients reporting increased nurse responsiveness to pain, nurse friendliness, and overall nursing care.[40] The culture surrounding ERAS focuses on including the patient as an active member of an engaged health care team dedicated to helping the patient recover, and seeing a positive impact on the patient's perception of his or her nursing care supports this cultural change with ERAS.

ADHERENCE

Thus far the article focused on individual components of ERAS contributing to improvements in quality metrics. However, it is important to emphasize that ERAS is a package of best practice recommendations throughout all phases of care, and an important component of its success is not individually selecting components to use, but implementing ERAS as a bundle. One of the limitations to many of the studies demonstrating improvement in ERAS is that it is not possible to demonstrate a causal relationship between an individual process measure and outcomes, as ERAS is often adopted as a bundle. There is strong evidence that suggests that high adherence to ERAS components is necessary to achieve quality improvement. The ERAS Compliance Group studied the impact of ERAS compliance on a large international cohort of patients and found a correlation between increasing ERAS compliance and decreased rates of complications (odds ratio [OR] 0.69, $P<.001$).[41] Similarly, using data from the National Surgical Quality Improvement Program (NSQIP), a higher adherence to ERAS was associated with fewer complications, faster recovery, and shorter LOS.[42] Poor ERAS adherence was also found to be independently predictive of readmission.[37]

Auditing ERAS adherence and understanding where there are failures is a key instrument that is paramount to successfully implementing ERAS. The feedback of this information to frontline providers is an essential step to keep all team members engaged and dedicated to improving the quality of patient care.[43] Implementation of ERAS should be an iterative process that is constantly undergoing improvements, and some components of flexibility with local adaptation may be necessary in order to successfully adopt ERAS.[43] Improving ERAS adherence also cannot be conducted in a silo. In order to have a high adherence to ERAS and successful implementation, transdisciplinary collaboration is necessary. Surgeons, anesthesiologists, nurses, and all health care providers need to work in a coordinated effort through all phases of care from preoperative care to postdischarge in order to improve ERAS adherence.[2] Studies have already shown that institutions that promoted safety culture were more successful at reducing HAIs.[44–46] Similarly, the safety culture of an institution is an important component of ERAS and contributes significantly to improving quality metrics.

SUMMARY

ERAS is an evidence-based protocol that aims to decrease the physiologic stress response to surgery and maintain postoperative physiologic function. This best practice bundle plays a significant role in improving surgical quality by impacting important quality metrics such as LOS, HAIs, readmissions, and patient experience. Adherence to ERAS as a collective bundle is more important than individual components in improving quality metrics, and this can only be achieved with data-driven information through auditing and interdisciplinary collaboration.

REFERENCES

1. Types of quality measures. 2018. Available at: http://www.ahrq.gov/professionals/quality-patient-safety/talkingquality/create/types.html. Accessed March 15, 2018.
2. Grant MC, Yang D, Wu CL, et al. Impact of enhanced recovery after surgery and fast track surgery pathways on healthcare-associated infections: results from a systematic review and meta-analysis. Ann Surg 2017;265(1):68–79.
3. Donabedian A. The quality of care. How can it be assessed? JAMA 1988;260(12):1743–8.
4. Greco M, Capretti G, Beretta L, et al. Enhanced recovery program in colorectal surgery: a meta-analysis of randomized controlled trials. World J Surg 2014;38(6):1531–41.
5. Varadhan KK, Neal KR, Dejong CH, et al. The enhanced recovery after surgery (ERAS) pathway for patients undergoing major elective open colorectal surgery: a meta-analysis of randomized controlled trials. Clin Nutr 2010;29(4):434–40.
6. Spanjersberg WR, Reurings J, Keus F, et al. Fast track surgery versus conventional recovery strategies for colorectal surgery. Cochrane Database Syst Rev 2011;(2):CD007635.
7. Varadhan KK, Lobo DN, Ljungqvist O. Enhanced recovery after surgery: the future of improving surgical care. Crit Care Clin 2010;26(3):527–47, x.
8. Hogan BV, Peter MB, Shenoy HG, et al. Surgery induced immunosuppression. Surgeon 2011;9(1):38–43.
9. Kadosawa T, Watabe A. The effects of surgery-induced immunosuppression and angiogenesis on tumour growth. Vet J 2015;205(2):175–9.
10. Scott MJ, Baldini G, Fearon KC, et al. Enhanced Recovery After Surgery (ERAS) for gastrointestinal surgery, part 1: pathophysiological considerations. Acta Anaesthesiol Scand 2015;59(10):1212–31.
11. Fearon KC, Ljungqvist O, Von Meyenfeldt M, et al. Enhanced recovery after surgery: a consensus review of clinical care for patients undergoing colonic resection. Clin Nutr 2005;24(3):466–77.
12. Jackson RS, Amdur RL, White JC, et al. Hyperglycemia is associated with increased risk of morbidity and mortality after colectomy for cancer. J Am Coll Surg 2012;214(1):68–80.
13. Svanfeldt M, Thorell A, Hausel J, et al. Effect of "preoperative" oral carbohydrate treatment on insulin action–a randomised cross-over unblinded study in healthy subjects. Clin Nutr 2005;24(5):815–21.
14. Gustafsson UO, Scott MJ, Schwenk W, et al. Guidelines for perioperative care in elective colonic surgery: Enhanced Recovery After Surgery (ERAS((R))) Society recommendations. World J Surg 2013;37(2):259–84.
15. Smith MD, McCall J, Plank L, et al. Preoperative carbohydrate treatment for enhancing recovery after elective surgery. Cochrane Database Syst Rev 2014;(8):CD009161.
16. Fabrizio AC, Grant MC, Siddiqui Z, et al. Is enhanced recovery enough for reducing 30-d readmissions after surgery? J Surg Res 2017;217:45–53.
17. Chatterjee S, Rudra A, Sengupta S. Current concepts in the management of postoperative nausea and vomiting. Anesthesiol Res Pract 2011;2011:748031.
18. Gan TJ, Meyer TA, Apfel CC, et al. Society for Ambulatory Anesthesia guidelines for the management of postoperative nausea and vomiting. Anesth Analg 2007;105(6):1615–28 [Table of contents].
19. Ljungqvist O. Insulin resistance and outcomes in surgery. J Clin Endocrinol Metab 2010;95(9):4217–9.

20. Guay J, Nishimori M, Kopp S. Epidural local anaesthetics versus opioid-based analgesic regimens for postoperative gastrointestinal paralysis, vomiting and pain after abdominal surgery. Cochrane Database Syst Rev 2016;(7):CD001893.

21. Marret E, Remy C, Bonnet F. Meta-analysis of epidural analgesia versus parenteral opioid analgesia after colorectal surgery. Br J Surg 2007;94(6):665–73.

22. Nisanevich V, Felsenstein I, Almogy G, et al. Effect of intraoperative fluid management on outcome after intraabdominal surgery. Anesthesiology 2005;103(1): 25–32.

23. Lobo DN, Bostock KA, Neal KR, et al. Effect of salt and water balance on recovery of gastrointestinal function after elective colonic resection: a randomised controlled trial. Lancet 2002;359(9320):1812–8.

24. Rahn DD, Mamik MM, Sanses TV, et al. Venous thromboembolism prophylaxis in gynecologic surgery: a systematic review. Obstet Gynecol 2011;118(5):1111–25.

25. Nelson R, Tse B, Edwards S. Systematic review of prophylactic nasogastric decompression after abdominal operations. Br J Surg 2005;92(6):673–80.

26. Semerjian A, Milbar N, Kates M, et al. Hospital charges and length of stay following radical cystectomy in the enhanced recovery after surgery era. Urology 2018;111:86–91.

27. Poggio JL. Perioperative strategies to prevent surgical-site infection. Clin Colon Rectal Surg 2013;26(3):168–73.

28. Nelson RL, Gladman E, Barbateskovic M. Antimicrobial prophylaxis for colorectal surgery. Cochrane Database Syst Rev 2014;(5):CD001181.

29. Nicholson A, Lowe MC, Parker J, et al. Systematic review and meta-analysis of enhanced recovery programmes in surgical patients. Br J Surg 2014;101(3): 172–88.

30. Popping DM, Elia N, Marret E, et al. Protective effects of epidural analgesia on pulmonary complications after abdominal and thoracic surgery: a meta-analysis. Arch Surg 2008;143(10):990–9 [discussion: 1000].

31. Levy BF, Scott MJ, Fawcett WJ, et al. Optimizing patient outcomes in laparoscopic surgery. Colorectal Dis 2011;13(Suppl 7):8–11.

32. Ballantyne JC, Carr DB, deFerranti S, et al. The comparative effects of postoperative analgesic therapies on pulmonary outcome: cumulative meta-analyses of randomized, controlled trials. Anesth Analg 1998;86(3):598–612.

33. Castelino T, Fiore JF Jr, Niculiseanu P, et al. The effect of early mobilization protocols on postoperative outcomes following abdominal and thoracic surgery: a systematic review. Surgery 2016;159(4):991–1003.

34. Ban KA, Gibbons MM, Ko CY, et al. Surgical technical evidence review for colorectal surgery conducted for the AHRQ safety program for improving surgical care and recovery. J Am Coll Surg 2017;225(4):548–57.e3.

35. Meddings J, Rogers MA, Macy M, et al. Systematic review and meta-analysis: reminder systems to reduce catheter-associated urinary tract infections and urinary catheter use in hospitalized patients. Clin Infect Dis 2010;51(5):550–60.

36. Merkow RP, Ju MH, Chung JW, et al. Underlying reasons associated with hospital readmission following surgery in the United States. JAMA 2015;313(5):483–95.

37. Francis NK, Mason J, Salib E, et al. Factors predicting 30-day readmission after laparoscopic colorectal cancer surgery within an enhanced recovery programme. Colorectal Dis 2015;17(7):O148–54.

38. Fredericks S, Yau T. Educational intervention reduces complications and rehospitalizations after heart surgery. West J Nurs Res 2013;35(10):1251–65.

39. Nagle D, Pare T, Keenan E, et al. Ileostomy pathway virtually eliminates readmissions for dehydration in new ostomates. Dis colon rectum 2012;55(12):1266–72.

40. Thiele RH, Rea KM, Turrentine FE, et al. Standardization of care: impact of an enhanced recovery protocol on length of stay, complications, and direct costs after colorectal surgery. J Am Coll Surg 2015;220(4):430–43.
41. ERAS Compliance Group. The impact of enhanced recovery protocol compliance on elective colorectal cancer resection: results from an international registry. Ann Surg 2015;261(6):1153–9.
42. Berian JR, Ban KA, Liu JB, et al. Adherence to enhanced recovery protocols in nsqip and association with colectomy outcomes. Ann Surg 2017. [Epub ahead of print].
43. Stone AB, Yuan CT, Rosen MA, et al. Barriers to and facilitators of implementing enhanced recovery pathways using an implementation framework: a systematic review. JAMA Surg 2018;153(3):270–9.
44. Wick EC, Hobson DB, Bennett JL, et al. Implementation of a surgical comprehensive unit-based safety program to reduce surgical site infections. J Am Coll Surg 2012;215(2):193–200.
45. Pronovost PJ, Berenholtz SM, Goeschel C, et al. Improving patient safety in intensive care units in Michigan. J Crit Care 2008;23(2):207–21.
46. Huang DT, Clermont G, Kong L, et al. Intensive care unit safety culture and outcomes: a US multicenter study. Int J Qual Health Care 2010;22(3):151–61.

Enhanced Recovery After Surgery and Its Effects on Patient Reported Outcomes

Jai Bikhchandani, MD

KEYWORDS

- Patient-reported outcomes • Global recovery • Recovery-specific quality of life

KEY POINTS

- Enhanced recovery programs have been successful in improving patient outcomes after colorectal surgery.
- Evaluation of enhanced recovery after surgery (ERAS) programs have primarily concentrated on early phase of recovery.
- Long-term recovery depends on patient-reported outcomes (PROs).
- Several instruments are available to measure PROs but need clinical application.
- Research on PROs is a must to expand the initial success of ERAS.

INTRODUCTION

The concept of fast-track surgery was first introduced in the early part of new millennium.[1] Later the term enhanced recovery after surgery (ERAS) was adapted, highlighting the significance of recovery at the heart of this important principle in perioperative care of surgical patients. Enhanced recovery protocols (ERPs) were developed with main goals of improving patient outcomes and accelerate recovery.[2] In the last 2 decades, the surgical community has achieved a good understanding of the factors that work against early recovery. Surgery of the gastrointestinal tract is associated with postoperative pain, stress, nausea, and vomiting. In addition, lack of early mobilization, use of narcotics, and absence of enteral intake leads to postoperative ileus. Ileus is a well-known precursor of delayed recovery after abdominal surgery. Recognition and avoidance of all these factors comprised the first step in enhanced recovery of these patients. However, discharge from the hospital is not synonymous with recovery. Postoperative recovery starts immediately after surgery but is complete only when patients attain their baseline status.[3] The pillars of recovery include physical, physiologic, symptomatic, functional, and emotional well-being.[4]

Disclosure: The author has nothing to disclose.
Department of Surgery, St Elizabeth Physicians, St Elizabeth Hospital, 20 Medical Village Drive, Suite 132, Edgewood, KT 41017, USA
E-mail address: jai.bikhchandani@stelizabeth.com

Surg Clin N Am 98 (2018) 1129–1135
https://doi.org/10.1016/j.suc.2018.07.002
0039-6109/18/© 2018 Elsevier Inc. All rights reserved.

Published data on ERAS programs have so far focused only on duration of hospital stay and complications. Researchers have largely ignored the global recovery and especially patient perspectives of outcomes after surgery.[5] This article narrates the importance of patient-reported outcomes (PROs) in evaluating success of ERAS programs. The purpose of this article is to emphasize the central role of PROs in ERPs.

PATIENT-REPORTED OUTCOMES

An outcome is an objective measure of the efficacy of an intervention.[6] Application of ERAS protocols has undoubtedly proven to result in early discharge of patients after colorectal surgery.[7] However, utilizing length of hospital stay as the sole indicator of recovery is flawed. Length of hospital stay depends on several confounding factors such as support structure at patient's home, patient's expectations, insurance status, and location of discharge (ie, home or a rehabilitation facility).[8] The surgical community has well recognized that a true recovery after surgery is not simply reflected by discharge from the hospital. Recovery is defined as "the act or process of becoming healthy after an illness or injury." The recovery period starts in the hospital but continues long after the patient is discharged from hospital, **Fig. 1**. Recovery after surgery may be categorized into three phases – early, intermediate, and late.[9] The patient's perception of recovery after surgery is the return to his or her baseline level prior to surgery, which may take several weeks to months.[10] This will encompass absence of any symptoms and the ability to perform usual activities or return to work. Hence, there is introduction of the term patient-reported outcomes (PROs). In literal words, PROs are defined as "any outcome reported directly by the patient".[11] The various multidimensional facets of recovery may best be assessed by patients themselves. Therefore, the natural process of evolution in assessment of ERAS must include PROs. To date, the most available data in the literature on success of ERAS have focused on in-hospital recovery process. There is paucity of literature on PROs in ERAS programs.[5] This may be due to the pressures from hospital systems and insurance providers to emphasize mostly on reducing length of hospital stay. This may also stem from the fact that implementation of ERAS protocols in an inpatient setting is much simpler compared with the effectiveness of providers in directly impacting patient care at home. In a meta-analysis of 38 studies evaluating ERPs for abdominal surgery between 2000 and 2013, 24 studies measured recovery outcomes within 30 days after surgery.[5] Only 2 studies reported outcomes at 60 days, and 1 study reported outcomes at 90 days.

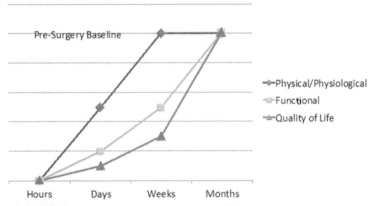

Fig. 1. Components and stages of recovery after surgery.

TOOLS TO MEASURE PATIENT-REPORTED OUTCOMES

PROs can be classified as

1. Symptoms reported by the patient
2. Functional status after surgery
3. Overall global health perception

SYMPTOM RECOVERY

Of all the PROs, symptom status may be the easiest to measure and report. Several authors have published on evaluation of ERAS programs based on symptom control.[12–15] Outcomes classified under symptom status are reflective of patient's perception of an abnormal physical or emotional state. Patient-reported symptoms may be pain, fatigue, nausea, vomiting, poor appetite, anxiety, or depression. Status of each of these symptoms should precisely be determined by the patient's reporting of his or her physical or emotional condition and not by an observer. A classical symptom after abdominal surgery is postoperative fatigue. The etiology may be multifactorial, but the impact on quality of life is often long, lasting from 1 to 3 months.[16] In the study by Zargar-Shoshtari and colleagues,[17] authors used the Identity-Consequence Fatigue Scale (ICFS) at several time intervals extending up to 60 days after surgery. The scale included 5 subcomponents – feelings of fatigue (5 questions), feelings of vigor (4 questions), impact on concentration (5 questions), impact on energy (6 questions), and instrumental activities of daily living (11 questions). The study concluded that the scores for the last 2 components, energy and activities of daily living, were significantly lower up to day 30 after surgery after ERAS program than conventional recovery protocols. From day 30 to day 60 after surgery, no statistical difference was noted. Similar outcomes have been reported by other authors.[18]

FUNCTIONAL RECOVERY

Functional recovery includes the patient's capacity to fulfill his or her physical, financial, and psychological commitments. The ability to ambulate at free will and perform baseline physical activity is an indicator of functional independence. Time to return to work and/or activities of leisure is also recorded to assess functional status (**Table 1**). Measures of activities of daily living (ADLs) and instrumental activities of daily living (IADLs) are useful in determining recovery.[19] An objective method of measuring patient's functional capacity after surgery is the 6-minute walk test. It is simply a measure of patient's exercise tolerance. The patient walks on a flat service for 6 minutes, at a pace that will tire him or her out. The total distance covered by the patient is measured in meters. This test has been validated as a measure of recovery 6 to 9 weeks after colorectal surgery.[20] The minimal clinically important difference for the 6-minute walk test has been estimated as 14 m.[21] Another tool to evaluate the level of physical activity in elderly patients after surgery is the Community Healthy Activities Model Program for Seniors (CHAMPS). The CHAMPS instrument is a 41-item questionnaire that essentially reports on the time spent performing a range of physical and social activities during the past week.[22] These activities are weighted appropriately to calculate the total caloric expenditure per week. Preliminary evidence supports the validity of CHAMPS to estimate recovery after cholecystectomy with the minimal clinically important difference estimated at 8 kcal/wk.[21] There are several advantages of objectively measuring physical performance. It does not completely depend on patient's perception and has objectivity to it. Serial measurements at sequential time intervals are feasible, and results can be applied clinically with confidence. A true quantification

Table 1 Tools or instruments currently available to measure patient-reported outcomes after surgery	
Functional Status	6-minute walk test
	Pedometer
	ADLs, IADLs
	Identity-Consequence Fatigue Scale
	CHAMPS score
	Hand grip
	Lower extremity test
	Return to work
	PROMIS
QOL instruments	SF36
	GIQOL
	Cleveland Clinic Global QOL
	EORTC QOL
	Quality of Recovery Score
	Postoperative Quality Recovery Scale
	Abdominal Surgery Impact Scale
	Surgical Recovery Scale

of postdischarge recovery can be obtained meaningfully. A recent tool developed by the National Institutes of Health (NIH) sponsored research called PROMIS (Patient-Reported Outcomes Measurement Information System).[23] The main aim of this system was to build an extensive item bank to evaluate physical function ranging from self-care to strenuous activities. Authors describe 4 domains to construct physical function that may be used for any disease process. These are IADLs, mobility or lower extremity function, back and neck (central function), and upper extremity function. The testing included 168 physical function items. PROMIS is one of the largest worldwide efforts to improve PRO measurement and accuracy.

The published data in literature on functional status after ERAS are scant. Assessment of patient mobilization by calculating time spent ambulating and/or pedometer recordings has been reported by few authors.[24,25] Jakobsen and colleagues[18] noted early functional return of patient after ERPs based on basic ADLs or IADLs. Benefit in cognitive function has also been described with accelerated recovery from ERPs.[26,27]

HEALTH PERCEPTION AND QUALITY OF LIFE

Perception of health and well-being is the most subjective of all PRO elements so far but probably one that influences patient recovery at the highest hierarchical level. Several indices have been designed to measure the quality of life after surgery (see **Table 1**). Commonly used questionnaires include Quality of Recovery Score (QoR 9, 15 40), World Health Organization Disability Assessment Schedule (WHODAS), Short Form 36 (SF36) Health Survey, and PROMIS. The best tool is one that measures the physical, mental, and social domains during the period of recovery. The tool should be validated and have responsiveness to surgical recovery.[28] SF-36 includes 36 items that can be divided into 8 domains assessing the physical (physical functioning, physical role, bodily pain), psychological (vitality, emotional role, and mental health), and social (social functioning) domains, as well as overall health (general health). Each domain is scored from 0 to 100. A recent study has validated SF-36 as measure of recovery after colorectal surgery.[29] However, the SF-36 scores were found to be similar after open versus laparoscopic surgery, suggesting a poor metric, as it needs to be able to differentiate the 2 different surgical approaches.[30] Such surveys have also been designed to be condition-specific like Gastrointestinal Quality of Life Index.[31] A systematic review article published on recovery-specific quality of life instruments concluded that there are 2 scales that merit further discussion.[32] The postdischarge surgical recovery scale records 15 criteria to measure recovery after ambulatory surgery. It includes activity, fatigue, work readiness, expectations, and health status.[33] The Quality of Recovery 40 score (QoR-40) looks at 5aspects of recovery: physical comfort, psychological support, physical independence, emotional state, and pain.[34] QoR-40 has been validated by scientific methods.[35] Subsequent to colorectal surgery, the QoR-40 scores reduce significantly on postoperative day 1 and recover to baseline on day 6 postoperatively.[36] Newer tools like Postoperative Quality Recovery Scale and Abdominal Surgery Impact Scale have also been reported.[9] PROMIS is a metric developed by NIH, which has been shown to be applicable after 15 different surgical operations, maintaining its validity and responsiveness.[37] Irrespective of the type of tool used, the PRO must be measured on day 1 after surgery, then at discharge, and ideally at postoperative days 30 and 90.[28]

SUMMARY

A perfect tool for PRO remains a matter of debate and research. The major limitations of the scales available currently include a high burden on a recovering patient for providing information as well as lack of measurement precision. The ultimate challenge is developing an instrument that must be comprehensive but at the same time simple enough to apply in a clinical setting. Striking a balance between these 2 objectives has been elusive to date. A logical start toward this goal will be to debate about the various instruments available. Designing a single tool encompassing the relevant observation points in several separate instruments needs ongoing research. Expert discussion is a must to reach a consensus on the core set of outcomes. Each domain of recovery should then be weighted based on its relative importance in the life of an individual patient with his or her specific needs.

CONCLUSIONS

ERAS programs decrease length of stay and postoperative complications and reduce hospitalization costs. Nevertheless, the impact of these programs on PROs, specifically functional recovery and QOL index, is not well known to date. Recording PROs is necessary in evaluating the effectiveness of ERAS pathways. Research on instruments that measure recovery-specific quality of life is the way to move forward in evaluating success of various enhanced recovery programs.

REFERENCES

1. Wimore DW, Kehlet H. Managements in fast track surgery. BMJ 2001;322:473–6.
2. Varadhan KK, Lobo DN, Ljungqvist O. Enhanced recovery after surgery: the future of improving surgical care. Crit Care Clin 2010;26:527–47.
3. Mayo NE, Feldman L, Scott S, et al. Impact of preoperative change in physical function on postoperative recovery: argument supporting prehabilitation for colorectal surgery. Surgery 2011;150:505–14.
4. Bowyer A, Jakobson J, Ljungqvist O, et al. A review of the scope and measurement of postoperative quality of recovery. Anesthesia 2014;69(11):1266–78.
5. Neville A, Lee L, Antonescu I, et al. Systematic review of outcomes used to evaluate enhanced recovery after surgery. Br J Surg 2014;101:159–70.

6. Macefield RC, Boulind CE, Blazeby JM. Selecting and measuring optimal outcomes for randomized controlled trials in surgery. Langenbecks Arch Surg 2014;399:263–72.

7. Lv L, Shao YF, Zhou YB. The enhanced recovery after surgery (ERAS) pathway for patients undergoing colorectal surgery: an update of meta-analysis of randomized controlled trials. Int J Colorectal Dis 2012;27:1549–54.

8. Maessen JM, Dejong CH, Kessels AG. Enhanced Recovery After Surgery (ERAS) Group. Length of stay: an inappropriate readout of the success of enhanced recovery programs. World J Surg 2008;32:971–5.

9. Feldman LS, Lee L, Fiore J Jr. What outcomes are important in the assessment of Enhanced recovery after surgery (ERAS) pathways? Can J Anaesth 2015;62: 120–30.

10. Blazeby JM, Soulsby M, Winstone K, et al. A qualitative evaluation of patient's experiences of an enhanced recovery programme for colorectal cancer. Colorectal Dis 2010;12:e236–42.

11. Washington AE, Lipstein SH. The patient-centered outcomes research institute – promoting better information, decisions, and health. N Engl J Med 2011;365:e31.

12. Delaney CP, Zutshi M, Senagore AJ, et al. Prospective, randomized, controlled trial between a pathway of controlled rehabilitation with early ambulation and diet and traditional postoperative care after laparotomy and intestinal resection. Dis Colon Rectum 2003;46:851–9.

13. Ionescu D, Iancu C, Ion D, et al. Implementing fast-track protocol for colorectal surgery: a prospective randomized clinical trial. World J Surg 2009;33:2433–8.

14. Jones C, Kelliher L, Dickinson M, et al. Randomized clinical trial on enhanced recovery versus standard care following open liver resection. Br J Surg 2013;100: 1015–24.

15. Raue W, Haase O, Junghans T, et al. 'Fast-track' multimodal rehabilitation program improves outcome after laparoscopic sigmoidectomy: a controlled prospective evaluation. Surg Endosc 2004;18:1463–8.

16. Paddison JS, Booth RJ, Fuchs D, et al. Peritoneal inflammation and fatigue experiences following colorectal surgery: a pilot study. Psychoneuroendocrinology 2008;33:446.

17. Zargar-Shostari K, Paddison J, Booth RJ, et al. A prospective study on the influence of a fast track program on postoperative fatigue and functional recovery after major colonic surgery. J Surg Res 2009;154:330–5.

18. Jakobsen DH, Sonne E, Andreason J, et al. Convalescence after colonic surgery with fast track vs conventional care. Colorectal Dis 2006;8:683.

19. Lawrence VA, Hazuda HP, Cornell JE, et al. Functional independence after major abdominal surgery in the elderly. J Am Coll Surg 2004;199:762–72.

20. Moriello C, Mayo NE, Feldman L, et al. Validating the six minute walk test as a measure of recovery after elective colon resection surgery. Arch Phys Med Rehabil 2008;89:1083–9.

21. Antonescu I, Scott S, Tran TT, et al. Measuring postoperative recovery: what are clinically meaningful differences? Surgery 2014;319:19–27.

22. Feldman LS, Kaneva P, Demyttenaere S, et al. Validation of a physical activity questionnaire (CHAMPS) as an indicator of postoperative recovery after laparoscopic cholecystectomy. Surgery 2009;146:31–9.

23. Rose M, Bjorner JB, Gandek B, et al. The PROMIS physical function item bank was calibrated to a standardized metric and shown to improve measurement efficiency. J Clin Epidemiol 2014;67:516–26.

24. Vlug MS, Wind J, Hollmann MW, et al. Laparoscopy in combination with fast track multimodal management is the best perioperative strategy in patients undergoing colonic surgery: a randomized clinical trial (LAFA-study). Ann Surg 2011;254: 868–75.
25. Henriksen MJ, Jensen MB, Hansen HV, et al. Enforced mobilization, early oral feeding, and balanced analgesia improve convalescence after colorectal surgery. Nutrition 2002;18:147–52.
26. Basse L, Raskov HH, Hjort Jakobsen D, et al. Accelerated postoperative recovery programme after colonic resection improves physical performance, pulmonary function and body composition. Br J Surg 2002;89:446–53.
27. Brazier JE, Harper R, Jones NM, et al. Validating the SF-36 health survey questionnaire: a new outcome measure for primary care. BMJ 1992;305:160–4.
28. Abola RE, Bennett-Guerrero E, Kent ML, et al. American society for enhanced recovery and perioperative quality initiative joint consensus statement on patient-reported outcomes in an enhanced recovery pathway. Anesth Analg 2018; 126(6):1874–82.
29. Antonescu I, Carli F, Mayo NE, et al. Validation of the SF-36 as a measure of postoperative recovery after colorectal surgery. Surg Endosc 2014;28(11):3168–78.
30. Lee L, Mata J, Augustin BR, et al. A comparison of the validity of two indirect utility instruments as measures of postoperative recovery. J Surg 2014;190:79–86.
31. Eypasch E, Williams JI, Wood-Dauphinee S, et al. Gastrointestinal quality of life index: development, validation and application of a new instrument. Br J Surg 1995;82:216–22.
32. Kluivers KB, Riphagen I, Vierhout ME, et al. Systematic review on recovery specific quality-of-life instruments. Surgery 2008;143:206–15.
33. Kleinbeck SV. Self-reported at-home postoperative recovery. Res Nurs Health 2000;23:461–72.
34. Myles PS, Weitkamp B, Jones K, et al. Validity and reliability of a postoperative quality of recovery score: the QoR-40. Br J Anaesth 2000;84:11–5.
35. Gornall BF, Myles PS, Smith CL, et al. Measurement of quality of recovery using the QoR-40: a quantitative systematic review. Br J Anaesth 2013;111:161–9.
36. Shida D, Wakamatsu K, Tanaka Y, et al. The postoperative patient-reported quality of recovery in colorectal cancer patients under enhanced recovery after surgery using QoR-40. BMC Cancer 2015;15:799–805.
37. Jones RS, Stukenborg GI. Patient-reported outcomes measurement system (PROMIS) use in surgical care: a scoping study. J Am Coll Surg 2017;224: 245–54.

Enhanced Recovery After Surgery
Economic Impact and Value

Lawrence Lee, MD, PhD[a],*, Liane S. Feldman, MD[b]

KEYWORDS

- Value • Costs • Economic evaluation • Organizational culture
- Patient-reported outcomes

KEY POINTS

- Value in health care is defined by the health outcomes achieved per dollar spent.
- Enhanced recovery pathways increase value by improving outcomes at similar or lower costs compared with traditional care.
- The economic literature is largely defined by colorectal ERPs, but there are increasing data to support its value in noncolorectal surgery.
- Long-term value of ERPs has yet to be fully defined.

INTRODUCTION

Health care spending is increasing at an unsustainable pace.[1] As of 2014, more than 17.1% of the US gross domestic product is devoted to health care.[2] Furthermore, the rate of increase in health spending outstrips that of the growth in gross domestic product (GDP).[1] In Canada, 10.4% of the GDP was spent on health care as of 2014, and this percentage has increased over the past few decades.[3] There is significant pressure from payers in all health care systems to improve quality and lower costs. It is within this context that an economic argument may be made for the adoption of enhanced recovery pathways (ERPs). It is commonly accepted that ERPs reduce costs by virtue of shorter duration of hospitalization and decreased complications.[4]

However, the impact of ERPs on cost may be more complex. First, the hospital days saved through an ERP are at the tail end of a hospital admission, which may not be resource intensive, because 40% of variable costs of a surgical admission occur

The authors have nothing to disclose.
[a] Department of Surgery, McGill University Health Centre, Steinberg-Bernstein Centre for Minimally Invasive Surgery and Innovation, 1001 Decarie Boulevard, DS1-3310, Montreal, Quebec H4A 3J1, Canada; [b] Division of General Surgery, McGill University Health Centre, Steinberg-Bernstein Centre for Minimally Invasive Surgery and Innovation, 1650 Cedar Avenue, L9-404, Montreal, Quebec H3G 1A4, Canada
* Corresponding author.
E-mail address: larry.lee@mcgill.ca

within the first 3 days.[5] Second, postoperative complications are the main cost driver of surgical admissions,[6] and randomized trials comparing enhanced recovery and traditional perioperative management have not unequivocally demonstrated a decrease in the incidence of postoperative complications.[7] As well, ERPs have no effect on the incidence of severe postoperative complications, that is, those that are most costly. Finally, care pathways may be associated with important design, implementation, and maintenance costs, which are not well described.[8] Surgeons leading ERPs should have a clear understanding of these issues in order to design effective programs for their specific contexts, including making a "business case" for implementation, which may require investments of resources initially. This article defines value in health care, summarizes the literature on the economic impact of ERPs, and discusses both the implementation costs and patient-centered benefits of ERPs in order to help surgeons advocate for the resources needed to implement and maintain an ERP.

LOWER COST OR HIGHER VALUE?

There is growing body of literature demonstrating improved surgical outcomes and lower costs with the use of ERPs for colorectal[9] as well as noncolorectal surgery.[10] Clearly, decreasing costs is of great importance, especially in the current health care environment. However, costs are only one side of the value equation. Michael Porter, an influential Harvard economist, has defined value in health care as "the health outcomes achieved per dollar spent."[11] Furthermore, Porter goes on to state that value "should always be defined around the customer." In other words, value is the attainment of the best outcomes that matter to the patient at the lowest cost. Therefore, a valuable intervention is one that either results in better outcomes at the same cost, the same outcomes at lower cost, or in the best-case scenario, better outcomes at lower cost.

Therefore, in order to improve the quality and cost-effectiveness of health care, 2 steps can be taken: decreasing or eliminating care that provides no benefit or offering interventions that provide good value for their cost.[12] ERPs potentially can fulfill both steps by eliminating surgical practices that may be harmful, such as perioperative starvation and prolonged postoperative bed rest, and replacing them with multiple evidence-based interventions within a single perioperative strategy that may reduce waste and variability and improve outcomes.

AVAILABLE ECONOMIC LITERATURE

There is ample published data demonstrating lower costs in favor of ERPs. A systematic review of economics evaluations of ERPs in colorectal surgery identified 10 studies that reported cost data.[9] There were 8 studies in which the ERP group had lower costs (**Table 1**). Although these data were promising, there were significant limitations with the available economic data. Most of the studies were performed from an institutional perspective and did not include societal costs such as productivity losses or caregiver burden. This was a significant limitation in that the postoperative trajectory after hospital discharge is poorly described. There were concerns that the burden of care would be transferred to the outpatient setting by discharging patients earlier and that the calculation of direct medical costs limited to the hospital inpatient setting would fail to capture these important costs. Moreover, the costing methodology and statistical analysis in these studies were poorly described (in the case of costing methodology) or mostly inappropriate (in the case of the method of statistical analysis).

In response to the limitations identified in the available economic evaluations of enhanced recovery pathways at that time, a formal cost-effectiveness analysis using

Table 1
Cost data reported in studies investigated enhanced recovery pathways versus conventional care in elective colorectal surgery

Study ID	Costs	ERP	CC	P/95% CI
Archibald et al,[51] 2011	Total hospital costs (direct + overhead)	US$ 11,662[a]	US$ 21,037[a]	P<.0001
Bosio et al,[52] 2007	Hospital direct costs	US$ 4993[a]	US$ 11,383[a]	P<.001
Folkerson et al,[53] 2005	Direct medical costs	DKK 17521	DKK 21340	N/A
	Indirect costs	DKK 18649	DKK 24134	
	Total costs	DKK 36170	DKK 45474	
Jurowich et al,[54] 2001	Hospital direct costs for the first 5 postoperative days	€ 1628	€ 2391	P = .001
Kariv et al,[55] 2007	Direct hospital costs	US$ 5692[b]	US$ 6672[b]	P = .001
King et al,[56] 2006	Total costs	£ 6545.29[a]	£ 7216.00[a]	95% CI: −1033.89–2433.53
	Indirect costs	£ 534.39[a]	£ 1061.50[a]	95% CI: 54.00–986.67
Ren et al,[57] 2012	Total costs of the procedure	CNY 15997[a]	CNY 17763[a]	P<.001
	Postoperative costs	CNY 3594[a]	CNY 5268[a]	P<.001
Sammour et al,[23] 2010	Total hospital costs (incl. protocol development and research fellow's salary)	NZ$ 16,052[a]	NZ$ 22,939[a]	Not reported
Stephen et al,[58] 2013	Total hospital costs (excl. surgeon's fees)	US$ 7070[a]	US$ 9310[a]	P = .002
Vlug et al,[59] 2011	Direct hospital costs (university hospitals)	€ 10,594 (lap)[b] € 12,805 (open)[b]	€ 11,967 (lap)[b] € 10,479 (open)[b]	P = .56
	Direct hospital costs (teaching hospitals)	€ 5768 (lap)[b] € 5497 (open)[b]	€ 6228 (lap)[b] € 5650 (open)[b]	P = .41

1 DKK = 0.1573 US$; 1 € = 1.2647 US$_{2010}, 1.3449 US$_{2011}; 1 CNY = 0.1506 USD; 1 NZD = 0.7260 USD; currency exchange rates at date of publication from www.xe.com.

Abbreviations: CNY, Chinese Yuan Renminbi; DKK, Danish Krone; NZ$, New Zealand dollars; US$, US dollars.

[a] Mean cost.

[b] Median cost.

Adapted from Lee L, Li C, Landry T, et al. A systematic review of economic evaluations of enhanced recovery pathways for colorectal surgery. Ann Surg 2014;259:673; with permission.

appropriate costing methodology and patient-reported outcomes was performed.[13] This study reported the costs from the Canadian institutional, health care system, and societal perspectives. A colorectal ERP was associated with decreased mean length of stay—9.8 days (standard deviation [SD] 12.2) versus 6.5 days (SD 6.0), P = .017—but no difference in 60-day postoperative complications. However, patients in the ERP group had less productivity losses, decreased caregiver burden, and lower outpatient resource utilization. There were also no differences in patient-reported outcomes between conventional care and enhanced recovery. ERP implementation and maintenance costs were estimated to be 153$ per patient ($1 CAN in 2013 = $0.81 US). Differences between ERP and conventional care did not reach statistical significance from the institutional (mean difference −1150 $CAN; 95% confidence interval [CI] −3487, 905) or health care system (mean difference −1602 $CAN; 95% CI −4050, 517) perspectives. However, total cost combining institutional, health care system, and societal costs was significantly lower in the ERP group (mean difference −2985 $CAN; 95% CI −5753, −373). The results of this study confirmed the "value" of enhanced recovery in that it lowered costs while maintaining the same quality outcomes. Another study reporting the economic outcomes after provincial-wide implementation of ERPs in Alberta, Canada demonstrated significant reductions in length of stay, complications, and readmissions in patients undergoing colorectal surgery, resulting in cost savings of $2806 to $5898 CAD per patient, despite a total implementation cost of $464,518 over the 2-year study period.[14]

However, it should be noted that these economic evaluations were performed from the Canadian perspective, and their costs may not be fully generalizable to the American system, given the difference in unit costs. In the systematic review of economic evaluations, there were 4 studies originating from the United States (see **Table 1**).[9] In all of these studies, ERPs were associated with decreased total direct hospital costs. None of these studies reported health care system or societal costs. Several additional US studies have been published since, but the results have been equivocal.[15–17] In the study with the more rigorous economic evaluation methodology, Miller and colleagues[15] did not identify a statistically significant difference in unadjusted (mean difference −2161 $US; 95% CI −6353, 2030) or adjusted (mean difference −1854; 95% CI −6072, 2363) medical costs between ERP and conventional care. However, this study did report that ERP was expected to generate cost savings in at least 85% of unadjusted and 82% of adjusted cost samples from bootstrap estimates. Two other studies, which have many of the same limitations that were identified in the initial systematic review of economic evaluations, reported lower direct medical costs in favor of ERP.[16,17] These data demonstrate the complexity of cost analyses; however, it should be noted that all of these studies support the notion of higher value care with ERP, with provision of better outcomes at the same cost, identical outcomes at the same cost, or better outcomes at lower costs.

Although most of the evidence originated from the colorectal surgery literature, there is increasing evidence to support the economic benefits of ERPs in noncolorectal surgery. The literature is too extensive to include every possible study in this review. **Table 2** demonstrates the systematic reviews investigating the effect of ERPs in noncolorectal surgery that include economic data. Although there is significant heterogeneity in the health care systems, patient populations, and study designs in each of the individual reviews, the overall weight of evidence has reported lower costs in favor of ERP.

IMPLEMENTATION COSTS

One of the important cost inputs in ERPs is the resources required to design, implement, and maintain these pathways. Although the up-front costs may seem prohibitively high,

Table 2
Cost data from systematic reviews of enhanced recovery pathways in noncolorectal surgery

Study	Population	Studies Reporting Cost Outcomes	Result/Effect Size
Beamish et al,[60] 2015	Gastric cancer surgery	10	Standardized mean difference −1.02; 95% CI −1.59, −0.45
Xiong et al,[61] 2016	Pancreatic resections	4	All 4 studies reporting lower costs with ERP
Wang et al,[62] 2017	Liver surgery	5	Standardized mean difference −0.31; 95% CI −0.47, −0.14
Miralpeix et al,[63] 2016	Gynecologic oncology	3	All 3 studies reporting lower costs with ERP
Fiore Jr et al,[64] 2016	Pulmonary resection	3	2 of 3 studies reporting lower costs with ERP
Galbraith et al,[65] 2018	Total joint arthroplasty	1	1 of 1 study reporting lower costs with ERP
Visioni et al,[10] 2018	Noncolorectal abdominal gastrointestinal surgery	8	Weighted mean difference −5109.1 $US (2016); 95% CI −5852.2, −4365.8

these overall costs are often more than recuperated based on the expected cost savings associated with ERPs, and they can also be amortized over the whole patient volume, and often results in negligible additional cost-per-patient. At our institution, a multidisciplinary group led by surgeon, anesthesiology, and nursing champions, and including other important allied health professionals (the Surgical Recovery [SuRe] workgroup) was formed to develop strategies that focus on patient recovery. This group has created ERPs for multiple resource heavy procedures across all specialties including colorectal, thoracic, urologic, hepatobiliary, bariatric, gynecologic, and orthopedic surgery. The breakdown of the costs associated with this workgroup is shown in **Table 3**. Although the overall cost seems high, there were 708 patients who were managed by an ERP developed by the SuRe workgroup, resulting in a mean cost per patient of $153 CAN. All of these pathways have been shown to be associated with important cost savings, which have more than compensated for the invested development/implementation costs.[18–20] Another study estimated that the implementation of ERP across an entire provincial hospital network required an investment of $528,459

Table 3
Breakdown of surgical recovery workgroup program costs over a 1-year period at the McGill University Health Center

	Cost (2013 CAN$)
Full-time ERP nurse coordinator (yearly salary)	81,225
Opportunity costs of ERP steering group (1 h/meeting × 26 meetings)	14,320
Nurse specialists and managers, nutritionist, physiotherapist, librarian, clinical leaders from surgery and anesthesia ($550 per meeting)	—
Patient education material (operating costs of work performed by a medical informatics center)	13,225
Total	108,770

Data from Lee L, Li C, Landry T, et al. A systematic review of economic evaluations of enhanced recovery pathways for colorectal surgery. Ann Surg 2014;259:670–6.

CAN over 2 years (2014 $CAN).[21] This study also estimated the "breakeven point," where the cost savings would be greater than the implementation costs, to be 93 to 236 cancer resections or 38 to 80 noncancer resections. It was further estimated based on these data that every $1 invested would result in $3.8 (range 2.4–5.1) in return.[22]

There have been few other studies that describe ERP implementation costs. Two studies from New Zealand[23] and Switzerland[24] reported implementation costs without detailed explanation as to what they included. One American study estimated the cost of ERP implementation at a quaternary academic medical center (**Table 4**).[25] This analysis included the costs of personnel, materials, equipment, and staff training. Furthermore, the costs were broken down based on an assumption that the upfront resources would be higher in the first year and gradually decrease as the ERP intervention is thoroughly implemented. The per-patient cost was also based on different case volumes. Based on their own experience of a mean 1.9-day decrease in length of stay, these implementation costs were recuperated across all analyzed case volumes (100, 250, and 500 cases per year). There are no studies in noncolorectal surgery. These data demonstrate that the upfront implementation costs are more than made up by the downstream cost savings and increases in value afforded by ERPs.

OUTCOMES THAT MATTER TO THE PATIENT—THE OTHER SIDE OF THE VALUE EQUATION

As mentioned earlier, Porter states that value "should always be defined around the customer." This definition has important implications for improving the quality and value of the health care delivered to the patient. "Valuable" interventions therefore are those that improve the outcomes that matter most to the patient. However, there are often significant discrepancies between the outcomes that health care providers consider to be important versus those that patients are the most concerned about.[26] If the goal of ERPs is truly to "enhance recovery," then recovery must be defined from the patient's point of view. Patients equate recovery to be the absence of symptoms and the return of their ability to perform activities as they could before surgery.[27] Recovery after surgery can be further defined as a multidimensional construct that follows a natural trajectory (**Fig. 1**) and is a comparative standard (ie, to a presurgical or a precondition baseline).[28]

However, most of the evidence detailing the clinical effectiveness of ERPs focuses on traditional audit measures such as length of stay and complications. Few studies investigate the impact of pathways on patient-reported outcomes.[29] Audit outcomes are proxy measures of recovery, because length of stay may be affected by external elements such as socioeconomic, cultural, and institutional factors,[30] and complications and mortality are relatively uncommon and often inconsistently measured.[31] These measures also emphasize the earliest period of recovery (the in-patient phase), whereas full recovery after major surgery often requires several months.[32]

The impact of ERPs on patient-centered outcome measures (PROMs) is less clear. A systematic review of the available PROMs in the context of recovery after surgery identified 22 different PROMs that were used by 35 different studies.[33] Most of these studies were of low methodological quality, and the PROMs used had limited validity evidence. Other studies that have used patient-centered outcomes (but not necessarily "patient-reported"—objective assessments of functional capacity such as hand-grip strength of cardiopulmonary exercise testing fall into this category) to compare ERP with conventional care have also demonstrated equivocal results.[34] Therefore, a more thorough evaluation of the true "value" of ERPs will require future studies to include more patient- and recovery-centric outcomes in addition to traditional audit measures.[35]

Table 4
Implementation costs at an American quaternary academic medical center

Costs	Annual No. of ERAS Cases		
	100	250	500
Implementation costs, $	10,000	10,000	10,000
Site visits/training course	0	73,700	135,839
Surgeon/anesthesia/nursing leadership time	0	25,000	50,000
Capita expenses, equipment, $			
Annual costs, $			
Personnel			
Project manager	100,875	100,875	126,094
Acute pain nurse	0	56,950	113,900
Preoperative support	0	28,475	56,950
Materials			
Education materials	2000	5000	10,000
Carbohydrate drinks/nutritional supplements	5000	12,500	25,000
Disposable materials related to fluid therapy monitor or other ERAS equipment	0	12,500	25,000
Total first-year costs, $	117,875	325,00	552,783
Annual maintenance costs, $	107,875	216,300	356,944
Cost per patient, year 1, $	1179	1300	1106
Cost per patient, non-year 1, $	1079	865	714

Adapted from Stone AB, Grant MC, Pio Roda C, et al. implementation costs of an enhanced recovery after surgery program in the united states: a financial model and sensitivity analysis based on experiences at a quaternary academic medical center. J Am Coll Surg 2016;222:221; with permission.

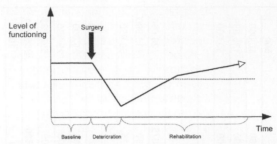

Fig. 1. Trajectory of postoperative recovery. (*From* Lee L, Tran T, Mayo NE, et al. What does it really mean to "recover" from an operation? Surgery 2013;155:212; with permission.)

ENHANCED RECOVERY AND MINIMALLY INVASIVE SURGERY—OPPORTUNITY FOR ADDED VALUE

There may be the impression that ERPs do not add additional benefit beyond laparoscopy. It is in this context that ERPs may further improve the quality and value of care delivered. Meta-analyses have shown that laparoscopic colectomy is associated with lower length of stay and complications compared with open surgery even within an ERP.[36,37] Programs such as the Society of American Gastrointestinal and Endoscopic Surgeons and Surgical Multimodal Accelerated Recovery Trajectory have been established to promote the uptake of ERPs to maximize the effects of Management Information System.[38]

ORGANIZATION VALUE—CHANGES IN CULTURE

Many of the ERP elements represent important departures from traditional perioperative care. Dogmas are intimately ingrained into surgical culture, which largely persist despite high-level evidence to the contrary.[39] One of the requirements of ERPs is multidisciplinary collaboration between specialties and the opening of lines of communication that may not have previously existed. This involves the breakdown of traditional silos of care, which may have important positive downstream effects in improving organizational culture.[40,41] Resistance to change has been identified as one of the major barriers to ERP implementation,[42] yet it is one that can be slowly broken down through enhanced multidisciplinary collaboration and communication, as well as support from hospital administration. Although it is difficult to accurately quantify this effect, higher levels of coordination and communication amongst services and staff have been associated with better outcomes.[43]

FUTURE DIRECTIONS

There may be other ways where ERPS may increase value. One aspect that has not been well investigated is the effect of ERPs on the ability of patients to undergo adjuvant therapies after surgery. It is postulated that ERPs, in reducing the negative impact of surgery, may allow for quicker return to intended oncologic therapy.[44,45] The more timely administration of adjuvant therapy may improve survival, especially for colorectal cancer.[46] Improvements in cancer care can significantly decrease overall long-term costs. Another question that remains unanswered is the proper valuation of having open beds as a result of ERPs (ie, the opposite of the opportunity cost of the beds occupied as a result of not using ERPs). Multiple randomized trials have consistently demonstrated that ERPs reduces length of stay.[7] As a result, there may be increased numbers of available hospital beds that can be directly attributable to ERPs. However, the downstream effects of this increased efficiency have not been clearly elucidated. On one hand, increased bed availability may increase operative capacity and decrease emergency department wait times. Reductions in operative wait time have been associated with improved long-term cancer survival and quality of life,[47,48] although this has not been consistently demonstrated for all neoplasms.[49] The true budgetary impact will depend on local factors, such as operational capacity and payment systems. Institutions that continuously function at full capacity will likely benefit the most from increased bed availability. Hospitals under prospective payment systems (ie, a predetermined amount based on a diagnosis) or global budgets may experience increased overall costs if available beds are occupied by high-cost acute cases instead of elective patients at the tail end of their surgical admission (which contribute minimally to hospital resource use and costs[5]). Conversely, revenue may also be increased due to higher capacity, because shorter length of stay may allow for higher turnover.[50] Future studies should account for all of these variables to determine the true costs and benefits of ERPs.

REFERENCES

1. Emanuel EJ. Where are the health care cost savings? JAMA 2012;307(1):39–40.
2. Health expenditure, total (% of GDP). 2018. Available at: http://data.worldbank.org/indicator/SH.XPD.TOTL.ZS. Accessed February 11, 2018.
3. Health expenditure, total (% of GDP). 2014. Available at: http://data.worldbank.org/indicator/SH.XPD.TOTL.ZS. Accessed July 14, 2014.
4. Kehlet H, Wilmore DW. Multimodal strategies to improve surgical outcome. Am J Surg 2002;183(6):630–41.
5. Taheri PA, Butz DA, Greenfield LJ. Length of stay has minimal impact on the cost of hospital admission. J Am Coll Surg 2000;191(2):123–30.
6. Dimick JB, Pronovost PJ, Cowan JA, et al. Complications and costs after high-risk surgery: where should we focus quality improvement initiatives? J Am Coll Surg 2003;196(5):671–8.
7. Zhuang CL, Ye XZ, Zhang XD, et al. Enhanced recovery after surgery programs versus traditional care for colorectal surgery: a meta-analysis of randomized controlled trials. Dis Colon Rectum 2013;56(5):667–78.
8. Lee L, Li C, Landry T, et al. A systematic review of economic evaluations of enhanced recovery pathways for colorectal surgery. Ann Surg 2013;261(5): e138.
9. Lee L, Li C, Landry T, et al. A systematic review of economic evaluations of enhanced recovery pathways for colorectal surgery. Ann Surg 2014;259(4): 670–6.
10. Visioni A, Shah R, Gabriel E, et al. Enhanced recovery after surgery for noncolorectal surgery?: a systematic review and meta-analysis of major abdominal surgery. Ann Surg 2018;267(1):57–65.
11. Porter ME. What is value in health care? N Engl J Med 2010;363(26):2477–81.
12. Owens DK, Qaseem A, Chou R, et al. Clinical guidelines committee of the American College of P. High-value, cost-conscious health care: concepts for clinicians to evaluate the benefits, harms, and costs of medical interventions. Ann Intern Med 2011;154(3):174–80.
13. Lee L, Mata J, Ghitulescu GA, et al. Cost-effectiveness of enhanced recovery versus conventional perioperative management for colorectal surgery. Ann Surg 2015;262(6):1026–33.

14. Nelson G, Kiyang LN, Crumley ET, et al. Implementation of enhanced recovery after surgery (ERAS) across a provincial healthcare system: the ERAS alberta colorectal surgery experience. World J Surg 2016;40(5):1092–103.

15. Miller TE, Thacker JK, White WD, et al. Reduced length of hospital stay in colorectal surgery after implementation of an enhanced recovery protocol. Anesth Analg 2014;118(5):1052–61.

16. Thiele RH, Rea KM, Turrentine FE, et al. Standardization of care: impact of an enhanced recovery protocol on length of stay, complications, and direct costs after colorectal surgery. J Am Coll Surg 2015;220(4):430–43.

17. Jung AD, Dhar VK, Hoehn RS, et al. Enhanced recovery after colorectal surgery: can we afford not to use it? J Am Coll Surg 2018;226(4):586–93.

18. Paci P, Madani A, Lee L, et al. Economic impact of an enhanced recovery pathway for lung resection. Ann Thorac Surg 2017;104(3):950–7.

19. Lee L, Li C, Robert N, et al. Economic impact of an enhanced recovery pathway for oesophagectomy. Br J Surg 2013;100(10):1326–34.

20. Abou-Haidar H, Abourbih S, Braganza D, et al. Enhanced recovery pathway for radical prostatectomy: implementation and evaluation in a universal healthcare system. Can Urol Assoc J 2014;8(11–12):418–23.

21. Nelson G, Kiyang LN, Chuck A, et al. Cost impact analysis of enhanced recovery after surgery program implementation in alberta colon cancer patients. Curr Oncol 2016;23(3):e221–7.

22. Thanh NX, Chuck AW, Wasylak T, et al. An economic evaluation of the enhanced recovery after surgery (ERAS) multisite implementation program for colorectal surgery in Alberta. Can J Surg 2016;59(6):415–21.

23. Sammour T, Zargar-Shoshtari K, Bhat A, et al. A programme of enhanced recovery after surgery (ERAS) is a cost-effective intervention in elective colonic surgery. N Z Med J 2010;123(1319):61–70.

24. Roulin D, Donadini A, Gander S, et al. Cost-effectiveness of the implementation of an enhanced recovery protocol for colorectal surgery. Br J Surg 2013;100(8):1108–14.

25. Stone AB, Grant MC, Pio Roda C, et al. Implementation costs of an enhanced recovery after surgery program in the united states: a financial model and sensitivity analysis based on experiences at a quaternary academic medical center. J Am Coll Surg 2016;222(3):219–25.

26. Lee L, Dumitra T, Fiore JF Jr, et al. How well are we measuring postoperative "recovery" after abdominal surgery? Qual Life Res 2015;24(11):2583–90.

27. Kleinbeck SV, Hoffart N. Outpatient recovery after laparoscopic cholecystectomy. AORN J 1994;60(3):394, 397-398, 401-2.

28. Lee L, Tran T, Mayo NE, et al. What does it really mean to "recover" from an operation? Surgery 2014;155(2):211–6.

29. Neville A, Lee L, Antonescu I, et al. Systematic review of outcomes used to evaluate enhanced recovery after surgery. Br J Surg 2014;101(3):159–70.

30. Perelman J, Closon MC. Impact of socioeconomic factors on in-patient length of stay and their consequences in per case hospital payment systems. J Health Serv Res Policy 2011;16(4):197–202.

31. Bruce J, Russell EM, Mollison J, et al. The measurement and monitoring of surgical adverse events. Health Technol Assess 2001;5(22):1–194.

32. Lawrence VA, Hazuda HP, Cornell JE, et al. Functional independence after major abdominal surgery in the elderly. J Am Coll Surg 2004;199(5):762–72.

33. Fiore JF Jr, Figueiredo S, Balvardi S, et al. How do we value postoperative recovery?: a systematic review of the measurement properties of patient-reported outcomes after abdominal surgery. Ann Surg 2018;267(4):656–69.

34. Feldman LS, Lee L, Fiore J Jr. What outcomes are important in the assessment of Enhanced Recovery After Surgery (ERAS) pathways? Can J Anaesth 2015;62(2): 120–30.
35. Wischmeyer PE, Carli F, Evans DC, et al. American society for enhanced recovery and perioperative quality initiative joint consensus statement on nutrition screening and therapy within a surgical enhanced recovery pathway. Anesth Analg 2018;126(6):1883–95.
36. Zhuang CL, Huang DD, Chen FF, et al. Laparoscopic versus open colorectal surgery within enhanced recovery after surgery programs: a systematic review and meta-analysis of randomized controlled trials. Surg Endosc 2015;29(8): 2091–100.
37. Spanjersberg WR, van Sambeeck JD, Bremers A, et al. Systematic review and meta-analysis for laparoscopic versus open colon surgery with or without an ERAS programme. Surg Endosc 2015;29(12):3443–53.
38. Feldman LS, Delaney CP. Laparoscopy plus enhanced recovery: optimizing the benefits of MIS through SAGES 'SMART' program. Surg Endosc 2014;28(5):1403–6.
39. Delaney CP, Senagore AJ, Gerkin TM, et al. Association of surgical care practices with length of stay and use of clinical protocols after elective bowel resection: results of a national survey. Am J Surg 2010;199(3):299–304 [discussion: 304].
40. Gotlib Conn L, McKenzie M, Pearsall EA, et al. Successful implementation of an enhanced recovery after surgery programme for elective colorectal surgery: a process evaluation of champions' experiences. Implement Sci 2015;10:99.
41. Lee L, Feldman LS. Improving surgical value and culture through enhanced recovery programs. JAMA Surg 2017;152(3):299–300.
42. Pearsall EA, Meghji Z, Pitzul KB, et al. A qualitative study to understand the barriers and enablers in implementing an enhanced recovery after surgery program. Ann Surg 2015;261(1):92–6.
43. Young GJ, Charns MP, Daley J, et al. Best practices for managing surgical services: the role of coordination. Health Care Manage Rev 1997;22(4):72–81.
44. Aloia TA, Zimmitti G, Conrad C, et al. Return to intended oncologic treatment (RIOT): a novel metric for evaluating the quality of oncosurgical therapy for malignancy. J Surg Oncol 2014;110(2):107–14.
45. Kim BJ, Caudle AS, Gottumukkala V, et al. The impact of postoperative complications on a timely return to intended oncologic Therapy (RIOT): the role of enhanced recovery in the cancer journey. Int Anesthesiol Clin 2016;54(4):e33–46.
46. Biagi JJ, Raphael MJ, Mackillop WJ, et al. Association between time to initiation of adjuvant chemotherapy and survival in colorectal cancer: a systematic review and meta-analysis. JAMA 2011;305(22):2335–42.
47. Smith EC, Ziogas A, Anton-Culver H. Delay in surgical treatment and survival after breast cancer diagnosis in young women by race/ethnicity. JAMA Surg 2013; 148(6):516–23.
48. Bourgade V, Drouin SJ, Yates DR, et al. Impact of the length of time between diagnosis and surgical removal of urologic neoplasms on survival. World J Urol 2014;32(2):475–9.
49. Amri R, Bordeianou LG, Sylla P, et al. Treatment delay in surgically-treated colon cancer: does it affect outcomes? Ann Surg Oncol 2014;21(12):3909–16.
50. Kahn KL, Keeler EB, Sherwood MJ, et al. Comparing outcomes of care before and after implementation of the DRG-based prospective payment system. JAMA 1990;264(15):1984–8.
51. Archibald LH, Ott MJ, Gale CM, et al. Enhanced recovery after colon surgery in a community hospital system. Dis Colon Rectum 2011;54(7):840–5.

52. Bosio RM, Smith BM, Aybar PS, et al. Implementation of laparoscopic colectomy with fast-track care in an academic medical center: benefits of a fully ascended learning curve and specialty expertise. Am J Surg 2007;193(3):413–5 [discussion: 415–6].

53. Folkerson J, Andreasen J, Basse L, et al. Health technology assessment of fast tracking colorectal surgery. 2005. English summary. Available at: http://www.sst.dk/publ/Publ2005/CEMTV/Acc_kolonkirurgi/Acc_kolonkir_patientforloeb.pdf. Accessed August 17, 2012.

54. Jurowich CF, Reibetanz J, Krajinovic K, et al. Cost analysis of the fast track concept in elective colonic surgery. Zentralbl Chir 2011;136(3):256–63 [in German].

55. Kariv Y, Delaney CP, Senagore AJ, et al. Clinical outcomes and cost analysis of a "fast track" postoperative care pathway for ileal pouch-anal anastomosis: a case control study. Dis Colon Rectum 2007;50(2):137–46.

56. King PM, Blazeby JM, Ewings P, et al. The influence of an enhanced recovery programme on clinical outcomes, costs and quality of life after surgery for colorectal cancer. Colorectal Dis 2006;8(6):506–13.

57. Ren L, Zhu D, Wei Y, et al. Enhanced Recovery After Surgery (ERAS) program attenuates stress and accelerates recovery in patients after radical resection for colorectal cancer: a prospective randomized controlled trial. World J Surg 2012;36(2):407–14.

58. Stephen AE, Berger DL. Shortened length of stay and hospital cost reduction with implementation of an accelerated clinical care pathway after elective colon resection. Surgery 2003;133(3):277–82.

59. Vlug MS, Wind J, Hollmann MW, et al. Laparoscopy in combination with fast track multimodal management is the best perioperative strategy in patients undergoing colonic surgery: a randomized clinical trial (LAFA-study). Ann Surg 2011;254(6):868–75.

60. Beamish AJ, Chan DS, Blake PA, et al. Systematic review and meta-analysis of enhanced recovery programmes in gastric cancer surgery. Int J Surg 2015;19:46–54.

61. Xiong J, Szatmary P, Huang W, et al. Enhanced recovery after surgery program in patients undergoing pancreaticoduodenectomy: a PRISMA-compliant systematic review and meta-analysis. Medicine (Baltimore) 2016;95(18):e3497.

62. Wang C, Zheng G, Zhang W, et al. Enhanced recovery after surgery programs for liver resection: a meta-analysis. J Gastrointest Surg 2017;21(3):472–86.

63. Miralpeix E, Nick AM, Meyer LA, et al. A call for new standard of care in perioperative gynecologic oncology practice: impact of enhanced recovery after surgery (ERAS) programs. Gynecol Oncol 2016;141(2):371–8.

64. Fiore JF Jr, Bejjani J, Conrad K, et al. Systematic review of the influence of enhanced recovery pathways in elective lung resection. J Thorac Cardiovasc Surg 2016;151(3):708–15.e6.

65. Galbraith AS, McGloughlin E, Cashman J. Enhanced recovery protocols in total joint arthroplasty: a review of the literature and their implementation. Ir J Med Sci 2018;187(1):97–109.

Preoperative Preparations for Enhanced Recovery After Surgery Programs
A Role for Prehabilitation

Gabriele Baldini, MD, MSc[a], Vanessa Ferreira, MSc[a,b],
Francesco Carli, MD, MPhil[a,*]

KEYWORDS

• ERAS • Preoperative assessment • Preoperative optimization • Prehabilitation

KEY POINTS

- Preoperative risk assessment, stratification, and optimization require a multidisciplinary approach, and should not be exclusively focused on patients' comorbidities.
- Preoperative risk assessment and stratification are valuable only if subsequent targeted optimization of patient care is allowed.
- Preoperative optimization requires time; early assessment of high-risk surgical patients is essential to facilitate appropriate optimization.
- The process of enhancing functional capacity of the individual to enable the patient to withstand the incoming surgical stressor has been termed prehabilitation.
- Multidisciplinary programs, such as prehabilitation, can address modifiable risk factors that may impact treatment outcomes.

INTRODUCTION

Almost 20 years ago, the concept of "fast track" was proposed with the understanding that it was necessary to revise surgical practice in view of the long hospital stay, high postoperative morbidity, and increasing health costs.[1,2] It was necessary to move forward from unimodal to multimodal interventions if surgical recovery was to be accelerated and morbidity reduced. In subsequent years, the Enhanced Recovery After Surgery (ERAS®) society was formed[3] with the intention to promote a multimodal and systematic approach to perioperative management and decrease postoperative

The authors have nothing to disclose.
[a] Department of Anesthesia, McGill University Health Centre, 1650 Cedar Avenue, Montreal, Québec H3G 1A4, Canada; [b] Department of Kinesiology and Physical Education, McGill University, 475 Pine Avenue West, Montreal, Québec H2W 1S4, Canada
* Corresponding author. Department of Anesthesia, McGill University, Montreal General Hospital, 1650 Cedar Avenue, Room D10.165.2, Montreal, Québec H3G 1A4, Canada.
E-mail address: franco.carli@mcgill.ca

Surg Clin N Am 98 (2018) 1149–1169
https://doi.org/10.1016/j.suc.2018.07.004
0039-6109/18/© 2018 Elsevier Inc. All rights reserved.

surgical.theclinics.com

morbidity as a result of standardized surgical care.[4] Surgeons began developing the infrastructure of ERAS and realized that it was necessary to involve other health providers if ERAS was going to achieve its goals. Clearly anesthesiologists, surgical nurses, physiotherapists, and nutritionists were needed to develop a sustainable program that would cover the whole surgical trajectory, from the preoperative clinic to hospital discharge. Many of the elements of the program, to name a few, carbohydrate drink, opioid-sparing analgesia, and intravenous fluid administration, are part of the anesthesia practice.[5,6] Knowledge on the underlying mechanisms of the stress response to surgery (endocrine, metabolic, and immunologic) and how to attenuate this response to prevent some of its negative effects (eg, increased oxygen consumption, cardiac demands, decreased gastrointestinal motility, pain) can facilitate the recovery process if integrated in the whole ERAS program. The anesthesiologist needs to be involved in various aspects of the ERAS program, for example, in the preoperative evaluation and optimization of preexisting organ dysfunction, the revision of fasting policy, the explanation to the patients and their families about the type of anesthesia and analgesia to be administered, the choice of perioperative care specific to the planned surgical procedure and with optimal intraoperative homeostasis and minimal organ dysfunction, thus facilitating rapid emergence and return of organ functions.

The implementation of procedure-specific ERAS protocols needs "champions" in various perioperative disciplines who need to meet regularly and review practice guidelines within the institution.[7] The anesthesiologist, as part of the group, must be aware of the continuous innovations in perioperative care and, as such, be flexible enough to make some changes in clinical practice and facilitate the implementation of the fast-track program. The present article has been written with the intention of addressing specific issues related to preoperative care, specifically in the context of ERAS programs. It provides evidence-based clinical approaches to best care starting in the preoperative clinic, where patients are informed about anesthesia and analgesia techniques, their health status is evaluated, and suggestions are given on how to improve functional capacity before surgery.

MINIMIZING THE SURGICAL STRESS RESPONSE: GENERAL CONSIDERATIONS

Surgery elicits a cascade of events that are broadly referred to as the stress response. This response is characterized by an increased release in neuroendocrine hormones and activation of the immune system via the upregulation of various cytokines. The combination of both a systemic inflammatory response and hypothalamic-sympathetic stimulation acts on target organs, including the brain, heart, muscle, and liver.[8] Central to the physiologic changes characterized by the inflammatory response is the relatively acute development of insulin resistance, which represents the main pathogenic factor modulating perioperative outcome, and it can be defined as an abnormal biological response to a normal concentration of insulin.[9] Insulin controls glucose, fat, and protein metabolism, and a change in insulin sensitivity by the cell, later the metabolic response. Hyperglycemia and protein breakdown represent the 2 main consequences of the low insulin sensitivity initiated by surgical insult.

Besides metabolic states such as cancer, obesity, diabetes, frailty, and sarcopenia, which characterize a preoperative state of insulin resistance, some intraoperative and postoperative elements that lead to a decrease in insulin sensitivity need to be mentioned: fasting, pain, bed rest, and fatigue.

As the pathophysiology of the stress response is multifactorial, it would make sense to plan a series of interventions aimed at attenuating the initiation of an insulin-resistant state. To that extent, the anesthesiologist, working as a team with the surgeon and the rest of the perioperative group, should consider a multimodal interventional strategy that could include the following: preoperative optimization and carbohydrate drink, neural de-afferentation, physiologic homeostasis, achievement of optimal nutritional and metabolic status, and enhancement of physical mobility.

PREOPERATIVE RISK ASSESSMENT, STRATIFICATION, AND CLINICAL OPTIMIZATION

Preoperative risk assessment and stratification are valuable only if subsequent, targeted optimization of patient care is allowed. The ultimate goal is to reduce postoperative morbidity and mortality, and facilitate surgical recovery. Surgery and organ-specific preoperative scoring systems can be integrated into preoperative clinical assessment to identify high-risk patients.[10] Similarly, biomarkers such as brain natriuretic peptide (BNP) and pro-BNP can also be used to estimate postoperative morbidity, further enhancing risk assessment and stratification.[11]

Poor preoperative functional status has been associated with increased morbidity and mortality, and prolonged surgical recovery.[12-15] Preoperative assessment of functional capacity can identify patients with poor functional status (low cardiopulmonary reserve) at high risk of developing postoperative complications and who are likely to benefit from preoperative prehabilitation and optimization.[16,17] It is commonly estimated by measuring metabolic equivalents or alternatively by using several functional tests, such as the 6-minute walking test (6MWT).[14-16]

Cardiopulmonary exercise testing (CPET) is a low-risk, noninvasive preoperative test that can more precisely and objectively determine functional capacity by measuring maximum oxygen consumption (VO_{2max}) and anaerobic threshold (AT). Peak oxygen consumption (VO_{2peak}), which is considered essentially similar to VO_{2max}, is more frequently used in clinical practice because surgical patients are not often able to achieve or are not sufficiently motivated to reach maximum oxygen uptake. AT should always be expressed as a percentage of the VO_{2max}, as oxygen consumption physiologically declines with aging.[18] Other parameters, such as pulmonary gas exchange and lactate, also can be obtained to interpret CPET main results. The results of the CPET can adequately inform perioperative physicians about the patient's ability to cope with the increased metabolic demand induced by surgical stress. Its use to stratify preoperative risk and identify high-risk patients requiring preoperative optimization, or to better allocate medical resources for the most vulnerable patients (ie, intensive care unit admission) has increased in the past 30 years. In fact, several observational studies in patients undergoing cardiovascular, thoracic, and abdominal surgery have shown that oxygen consumption at the AT less than 10 to 11 mL/kg per minute or VO_{2peak} less than 15 mL/kg per minute[19] can identify patients at high risk of developing postoperative complications.[20-26] Similarly, reduced AT has also been associated with increased mortality in the immediate postoperative period.[27-32] Moreover, in a large prospective observational study (n = 1725), the addition of CPET variables derived at AT improved the accuracy of other clinical (vital capacity), demographic (gender), and surgical variables (type of surgery) predicting long-term survival after thoraco-abdominal surgery[33] (**Table 1**). Candidates for CPET can be identified based on the presence of clinical risk factors or based on the results of functional tests, such as the 6MWT.[14] Interpretation of its results requires a team of experts and trained caregivers, as determination of AT can be influenced by several factors and therefore produce misleading results.[18] Variation of CPET protocols, interobserver and intraobserver variation of CPET results, learning effect, and preoperative

Table 1
Preoperative CPET and association with postoperative outcomes

Study	Type of Study, n	Surgery	Preoperative CPET Variables	Postoperative Outcome	Clinically Relevant Results
Older et al,[27] 1993	Observational, 187	Major abdominal Age >60 y	AT	Mortality	Higher mortality (18% vs 0.8%) if AT <11 mL/kg/min
Older et al,[28] 1999	Interventional, 548	Intra-abdominal Age >60 y	AT	Mortality	11% mortality[a] in patients with AT < 15 mL/kg/min 0% mortality in patients with AT > 14 mL/kg/min
McCullough, et al,[20] 2006	Observational, 109	Laparoscopic RGB	VO2max	Morbidity	VO2max <16 mL/kg/min
Snowden et al,[21] 2010	Major abdominal (colorectal excluded)	AT	Morbidity LOS	Morbidity LOS	AT <10.2 mL/kg/min predicted >1 postoperative complications
Wilson et al,[29] 2010	Observational, 847	Elective colorectal, nephrectomy, or cystectomy Age >59 y	AT	Mortality	AT <10.9 mL/kg/min Overall: RR = 6.8, 95% CI 1.6–29.5) Patients without cardiac risk factors RR = 10.0, 95% CI 1.7–61.0
West et al,[22] 2014	Observational, 136	Colorectal surgery	AT VO2peak VE/VCO2[b]	Morbidity	Patients with at least 1 complication had a median AT = 9.9 mL/kg/min; VO2peak = 15.2 mL/kg/min; VE/VCO2 = 31.3 mL/kg/min, significantly lower than patients without complications (P < .005)

Study	Study type, No.	Procedure	CPET variable	Outcome	Results
Grant et al,[30] 2015	Observational, 506	EVAR	AT VO_{2peak} VE/VCO2[b] at AT > 42	1 and 3-y survival	VE/VCO2 at AT > 42, and VO_{2peak} < 15 mL/kg/min independently predict reduced survival; reduction in AT independently predicts complications
Carlisle et al,[31] 2007	Observational, 130	Open AAA repair	AT VE/VCO2	Midterm survival	AT HR = 0·84 (0·72–0·98) VE/VCO2 HR = 1.13 (95% CI 1.07–1.19)
Epstein et al,[32] 2004	Observational, 59	Liver transplantation	VO_{2peak} AT	Mortality	AT independently associated with mortality (adjusted OR = 14.1, P = .03)
Forshaw et al,[23] 2008	Observational, 78	Esophagectomy	AT VO_{2peak}	Morbidity	VO_{2peak} lower in patients with cardiopulmonary complications (19.2 mL/kg/min vs 21.4 mL/kg/min, P = 04)
Nagamatsu et al,[24] 2001	Observational, 91	Esophagectomy	VO_{2max} AT	Morbidity	VO_{2max} independently predicts postoperative complications (P = .001)
Nugent et al,[25] 1998	Observational, 30	Open AAA repair	VO_{2peak}	Morbidity	VO_{2peak} < 20 mL/kg/min in 70% patients who had complications vs 50% in those who had not

Abbreviations: AAA, abdominal aortic aneurysm; AT, anaerobic threshold; CI, confidence interval; CPET, cardiopulmonary exercise training; EVAR, endovascular abdominal aortic aneurism repair; HR, hazard ratio; LOS, length of stay; OR, odds ratio; RGB, Roux-en-Y gastric bypass; RR, relative risk of non-survival; VO_{2max}, maximum oxygen consumption; VO_{2peak}, peak oxygen consumption.

[a] Estimated by the reported figure.

[b] Ventilatory equivalent for CO_2.

medications (beta-blockers) can all affect the measurement of AT.[18] Awareness of such pitfalls is crucial to avoid taking wrong preoperative clinical decisions.

Reestablishing baseline levels (eg, after neoadjuvant chemo-radiation therapy), or even improving baseline functional capacity before surgery, can be particularly important to increase physiologic reserve, to attenuate the impact of surgical stress, and to ensure a rapid and safe recovery. Interestingly, the results of a pilot study showed that the response to neo-adjuvant chemo-radiation therapy in patients treated with an intense exercise program before surgery was more effective than in patients in the control group, as demonstrated by a better MRI tumor staging 9 weeks after surgery.[34]

Surgical patients are frequently anemic preoperatively. In patients undergoing noncardiac surgery, the prevalence of preoperative anemia is estimated at approximately 30%[35] and has been reported as high as 90% in oncologic patients.[36] The pathogenesis of preoperative anemia is multifactorial: iron deficiency, chronic inflammation, myelosuppression, and renal impairment are the most common causes of anemia in surgical patients. Several studies have demonstrated an association between preoperative anemia and adverse outcomes.[37] Considering that allogeneic blood transfusion also has been independently associated with increased morbidity, mortality, and worse oncologic outcomes,[37] early identification of anemic patients is crucial to facilitate optimization of hemoglobin levels before surgery, without necessarily relying on blood transfusion. However, allogeneic blood transfusions remain essential to rapidly restore physiologic hemoglobin levels of severely anemic patients. Correction of preoperative anemia takes time and it can require a multidisciplinary approach, including anesthesiology and internists, hematology, transfusion medicine, gastroenterology, and education of all caregivers responsible for surgical patients.[38,39] Despite studies consistently demonstrating an association between preoperative anemia and postoperative morbidity and mortality, evidence suggesting that correcting preoperative hemoglobin levels improves postoperative outcomes is scarce.[39–41] A recent large prospective multicenter cohort study including 129,719 surgical patients showed that implementation of a patient blood management program, combining multidisciplinary perioperative interventions to increase and preserve autologous erythrocyte volume, is feasible and safe, and it significantly reduces the number of red blood cells and the incidence of acute renal failure.[42] Finally, it must be considered that anemic patients struggle to be compliant with exercise programs because of generalized fatigue. Optimizing preoperative hemoglobin levels in such patients might be beneficial to increase adherence to prehabilitation.

Preoperative screening of nutritional risk, and preoperative nutritional assessment and optimization also should be part of preoperative evaluation, as poor nutritional status not only increases the risk of postoperative complications,[43,44] but it has also been associated with worse oncologic outcomes.[45] It has been reported that the prevalence of malnutrition in patients with cancer ranges between 20% and 70%, depending on patient age and on the type and stage of cancer.[46] In fact, loss of appetite, metabolic rearrangements induced by the tumor, nausea and vomiting associated with oncologic treatments, and physical limitations induced by the cancer (eg, gastrointestinal obstruction) can significantly compromise the nutritional status of oncologic patients.[44] Identification of malnourished patients or patients at nutritional risk is crucial, and several validated scoring systems and questionnaires can be used.[44] Surgical patients should be routinely screened for malnutrition, and nutritional interventions should be given to malnourished patients and patients at nutritional risk. Preoperative nutritional interventions, preferably using the enteral route, should be given for at least 7 days before surgery.[44] If the energy and nutrient requirements cannot be met by oral and enteral intake alone (<50% of caloric requirement), parenteral nutrition also should be initiated. In patients in whom enteral nutrition is contraindicated or not feasible (eg, bowel obstruction), parenteral nutrition should be commenced as soon as possible.[44] Nutritional supplementation might be recommended in non-malnourished patients, as it helps to prevent serious postoperative complications and to maintain nutrition during the postoperative period.[44,47] Although the role of immunonutrition is controversial, guidelines recommend the administration of specific formula enriched with immunonutrients in malnourished patients undergoing major cancer surgery.[44] It is well established that optimizing nutritional status of malnourished patients scheduled for surgery decreases postoperative complications[44,48]; however, the impact of nutritional interventions on oncologic outcomes remains to be further investigated. A small randomized clinical trial suggested that in surgical patients with head and neck cancer, preoperative and postoperative arginine supplementation reduced the infection rate and impact on survival.[49] Moreover, a large retrospective study conducted in the context of an ERAS program demonstrated that high adherence to ERAS interventions, including those to optimize the nutritional status of malnourished patients with colorectal cancer scheduled for surgery, was associated with an improvement of cancer-specific survival and a reduction of cancer-specific death by 42% (hazard ratio = 0.58, 95% confidence interval = 0.39–0.88).[50]

The preoperative period also should be considered as an opportunity to change unhealthy lifestyle behaviors, such as smoking, and improve long-term outcomes.[51] Preoperative intense smoking cessation programs, including nicotine replacement therapy and patient counseling, have been associated with fewer postoperative infectious complications and long-term smoking abstinence, but only if initiated 4 weeks before surgery.[52] Alternatively, shorter interventions, such as preoperative treatment with Varenicline in association with patient counseling, can be prescribed.[53]

Psychological evaluation also should be part of the preoperative assessment, especially for oncologic patients. Despite animal and clinical trials suggesting that psychological stress can potentiate the stress response associated with surgery and facilitate cancer metastasis, implementation of psychological strategies in patients with cancer have failed to improve oncologic outcomes.[51] Nevertheless, it has been suggested that intervening throughout the entire perioperative period might be more beneficial than treating these patients solely in the postoperative period.[51] Moreover, psychological optimization has been associated with better postoperative analgesia and less analgesic consumption.[54]

Finally, with an aging population that continues to grow, elderly oncologic patients are more frequently scheduled for surgery. In this population, risk assessment is complex and it should require a multidisciplinary approach. It should not only include the risk associated with concomitant comorbidities, but also the risk of postoperative delirium, cognitive impairment, risk of falls, and the patient's frailty.[55]

FACILITATORS, BARRIERS, CHALLENGES

Optimal preoperative risk assessment, stratification, and optimization require a multidisciplinary approach, including anesthesiologists, internists, nurses, nutritionists, and smoking cessation facilitators. Implementation of a multidisciplinary preoperative clinic can facilitate risk assessment and optimization, and it has been associated with a reduction in postoperative morbidity and mortality.[56] It is also a great opportunity to inform patients about their surgical journey, the enhanced perioperative pathway, and seek for anesthesia consent after detailed discussion of most common anesthesia techniques.

Preoperative optimization might be challenging, as patients are frequently scheduled to be operated within a few weeks of the surgical diagnosis, leaving little or no time to optimize high-risk patients. This approach leaves high preoperative risk unmodified. This is particularly true for patients with cancer who in addition to the risk associated with their concomitant diseases[11,57–61] have specific oncologic conditions that further increase their risk of developing postoperative complications[62] (**Fig. 1**). If on the one hand it is commonly believed that immediate surgical resection of the tumor is crucial to avoid cancer recurrence and dissemination, on the other hand it must also be acknowledged that operating nonoptimized, high-risk patients significantly increases the risk of morbidity and mortality.[63] The decision to eventually delay surgery to optimize high-risk patients should consider the biology of the tumor, tumor staging, patients' physical status, and the effectiveness of preoperative interventions aimed at reducing the surgical risk. Evidence suggesting that postponing elective oncologic procedures to permit preoperative optimization of high-risk patients does not negatively affect oncologic outcomes is lacking, but urgently needed. In the meantime, preoperative evaluation of high-risk oncologic patients should be scheduled as early as possible, to permit medical and functional optimization.

PREHABILITATION TO INCREASE FUNCTIONAL CAPACITY BEFORE SURGERY
Surgery and Recovery

There is strong evidence that many of the negative immediate effects of surgery and cancer treatment, such as pain, fatigue, fluid overload, and weakness, can be

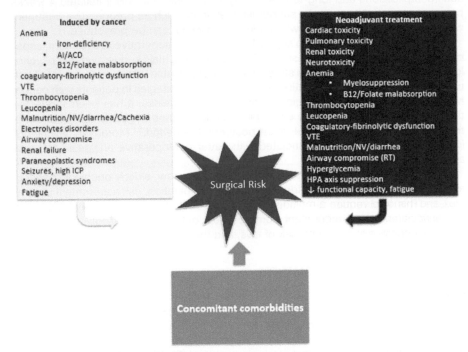

Fig. 1. Preoperative determinants of surgical risk in oncologic surgical patients. Surgery. related factors are not reported. AI/ACD, anemia if inflammation/anemia of chronic diseases; HPA, hypothalamic, pituitary, adrenal; ICP, intracranial pressure; NV, nausea and vomiting; RT, radiation therapy; VTE, venous thrombus embolism.

attenuated if adequate interventions are carried out, thus facilitating a faster recovery and early hospital discharge.[64] It would be of practical benefit if ways of improving postsurgery physical function and quality of life could be identified. Unfortunately, efforts are made to improve the recovery process by intervening in the postoperative period, which is not the most opportune time to introduce interventions to accelerate recovery because patients are tired, depressed, and anxious about further treatment they might receive. The preoperative period may be, then, a more emotionally opportune time to intervene while patients are scheduled for extra tests, and are anxiously waiting for surgery.

Increasing Functional Capacity by Prehabilitation

In the preoperative assessment of patients presenting for surgery, functional capacity is measured to estimate surgical risk and the need for intervention. As previously described, low functional capacity is correlated with an increase in postoperative complications.[21,29,65] It would therefore make sense if functional capacity can be increased before surgery, thus attenuating the postoperative risk. The process of enhancing functional capacity of the individual to enable him or her to withstand the incoming surgical stressor has been termed prehabilitation.[66,67] The concept of prehabilitation began in the orthopedic population (hip and knee arthroplasty) in which the impact of physical activity/exercise on postoperative outcome following surgery was addressed. The study of prehabilitation has since expanded to cardiac, vascular, and abdominal surgery. There is increasing evidence from the literature that preoperative exercise enhances physiologic reserve before and after surgery, with earlier return to baseline values. Recent systematic reviews reported that compared with standard care, prehabilitation reduced length of hospital stay and postoperative complication rate, and improved postoperative pain and physical and physiologic function[68–70]; however, interventions based on exercise alone may not be sufficient to enhance functional capacity. A randomized controlled trial in 112 patients undergoing colorectal surgery who received either a sham intervention of basic recommendations to walk daily and perform breathing exercises (control group) or a home-based high-intensity training program (aerobic and resistance exercises) demonstrated that patients in the control group experienced greater improvements in functional walking capacity compared with the intervention group.[71] Compliance to the high-intensity training program was only 16%, indicating that the prescribed exercise could not be maintained. Thus, a multimodal prehabilitation program has been recently proposed that includes structured aerobic and resistance exercise that is complemented by nutritional counseling, protein supplementation, and relaxation strategies to attenuate anxiety. This intervention is based on the understanding of the synergistic effect achieved by exercise in conjunction with protein administration to maximize muscle protein synthesis and therefore increase muscle strength.[72] The multimodal intervention was conducted in a pilot study[73] followed by a randomized controlled trial[74] in 164 patients undergoing colorectal resection. Results showed that more than 80% of patients were able to return to preoperative functional capacity by 8 weeks after surgery compared with only 40% in the control group.

Exercise Before Surgery

There is overwhelming evidence on the role of exercise in disease prevention, in fact, regular exercise has been shown to decrease the incidence of ischemic heart disease, diabetes, stroke, cancer progression, and fractures in the elderly. These achievements are a result of the various benefits associated with participating in regular physical activity, such as improvements in aerobic capacity, increased ratio of lean body mass to body fat, antioxidant capacity, better insulin sensitivity, and decreased sympathetic hyperactivity. Therefore, engaging surgical patients in physical activity and structured exercise programs to improve functional capacity in preparation for surgery is worth exploring; however, the literature on surgical prehabilitation is limited.

The traditional approach to the preoperative timeframe is to encourage rest to best prepare the patient for the upcoming surgery and initiate exercise only postoperatively as rehabilitation. However, bed rest has deleterious effects on lean muscle mass, physical function, lower extremity strength/power, aerobic capacity, and homeostasis.[75–77] Contrary to this standard, an exercise-mediated intervention initiated preoperatively, such as prehabilitation, has shown to result in greater improvements in functional walking capacity throughout the whole perioperative period when compared with rehabilitation started after surgery[72] (**Fig. 2**). These improvements are even more meaningful in patients with poorer fitness levels. Patients with lower baseline walking capacity experienced greater improvements in functional status with prehabilitation compared with patients with higher fitness.[78] However, such programs are only as effective as the adherence to them. The most commonly reported barriers for patients with cancer enrolled in a supervised prehabilitation program were parking (finding and paying for parking), transportation, and time.[79] Last, patient safety is a priority when participating in an exercise program. Prehabilitation programs have shown to be safe, even for elderly patients, whether they were delivered as home-based or center-based programs.[34] However, exercise performed under the supervision of an exercise specialist provides an added safety benefit. Careful considerations must be taken when developing a prehabilitation program to maximize adherence and ensure safety, as they can significantly influence the effectiveness of the program.

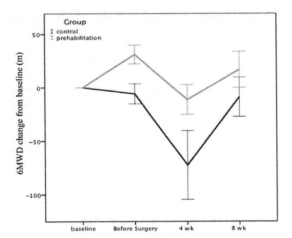

Fig. 2. The trajectory of the changes in functional capacity through the perioperative period in the prehabilitation and the control groups. Patients in the prehabilitation group received the trimodal intervention (exercise, nutrition, and relaxation strategies) before surgery. Patients in the control group started the same trimodal intervention (rehabilitation) after surgery. Error bars represent the 95% confidence interval. 6MWD = 6-minute walk distance. (*From* Minnella EM, Bousquet-Dion G, Awasthi R, et al. Multimodal prehabilitation improves functional capacity before and after colorectal surgery for cancer: a 5-year research experience. Acta Oncol 2017;56(2):298; with permission.)

Exercise Prescription

The term exercise refers to regular physical activity that is planned and structured for the specific goal of improving or maintaining fitness.[80] To better prepare for surgery, a preoperative exercise program should incorporate the 4 main types of exercise training: aerobic, strength, balance, and flexibility. Aerobic training stimulates the cardiovascular system by augmenting ventilator capacity and heart rate. It has been shown to be effective in improving physical fitness in patients awaiting intracavity surgery,[81] as well as improving cancer-related fatigue and quality of life.[82] An inexpensive and easy-to-perform test to assess functional exercise capacity is the 6MWT. The 6MWT has been validated in patients with cancer and is commonly used as a predictor for postoperative morbidity and mortality; however, it also can be used in the prescription of aerobic training, such as a walking program.[83]

Strength training focuses on resistance exercises to induce muscular contractions, promoting muscle anabolism, mass, and strength. Increasing lean muscle mass before surgery is key, given that muscle wasting is a typical phenomenon resulting from the catabolic effects of surgery in addition to the progressive muscle loss associated with aging.[84,85] Emphasis should be placed on exercises that reflect functional movements of daily living (ie, standing up from a seated position, which predominantly uses quadriceps muscular strength). Strengthening such muscles is particularly important for older adults, as they are associated with fall risk. Functional fitness tests, such as the 30-second sit-to-stand and arm curl test, can be used to predict muscular strength of the lower and upper limbs, respectively.[86]

In addition to aerobic and strength training, it is equally important to consider balance and flexibility training as necessary components of exercise prescription, particularly for the elderly population that is at an increased risk for falls and has limited range of motion. Given the relatively condensed period in which prehabilitation is being performed, careful monitoring of the program is of importance.

Just as the prescription of medication requires a specific dosage, delivery form, and frequency, the prescription of exercise should be given the same degree of precision. According to the American College of Sports Medicine (ACSM), the prescription of an exercise program should be tailored to the needs and desired outcomes of the patient by using the FITT principle[87]: frequency, intensity, timing, and type. Frequency refers to how often, usually the number of days per week, the patient should engage in exercise. The ACSM recommends healthy individuals to engage in aerobic training 3 to 5 days per week, resistance training 2 to 3 days per week, and flexibility/balance training most days of the week, especially following resistance training.[87] Intensity is the level of exertion experienced during exercise, which can be monitored using the 6 to 20 Borg scale (**Fig. 3**), a well-validated index of perceived exertion[88,89] or by tracking heart rate. The intensity recommended for aerobic exercise is moderate to vigorous intensity that is equivalent to 12 to 16 on the Borg scale (somewhat hard to hard) or a target heart rate between 40% and 85% of heart rate reserve (HRR).[87] Target heart rate is calculated by the Karvonen method: target heart rate = {[(220 − age) − resting heart rate] × percent intensity} + resting heart rate. For resistance exercise, 50% to 70% of 1 repetition maximum (maximal weight that can be lifted 1 time) in 2 or 3 sets with 8 to 12 repetitions per set has shown to be effective.[87] Time refers to the duration of the exercise, which should be between 20 and 60 minutes for aerobic training and 30 minutes for resistance training.[87] For flexibility training, each stretch should be held for 15 to 30 seconds and repeated 2 to 4 times.[87] Finally, type refers to exercise modality and can be any of the 4 types of exercise mentioned previously. A guide for a FITT exercise prescription is shown in **Table 2**.

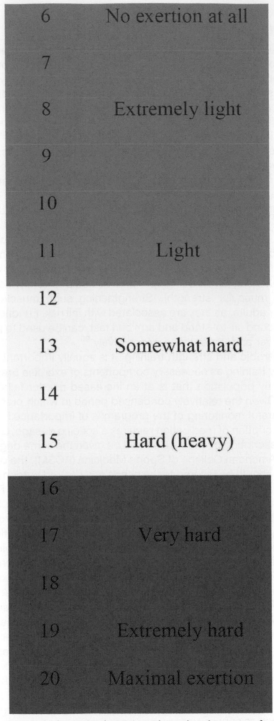

Fig. 3. The Borg scale rating of perceived exertion. The scale values range from 6 to 20 and can be used to denote heart rates ranging from 60 to 200 beats per minute. Moderate intensity exercise registers 11 to 14, whereas vigorous exercise rates 15 or higher on the Borg scale. (*Data from* Borg G. Perceived exertion as an indicator of somatic stress. Scand J Rehabil Med 1970;2(2):92–8.)

Table 2
FITT exercise prescription

FITT Principle Components	Frequency	Intensity	Time	Type
Aerobic training	3–5 d per wk.	Moderate: 40%–60% of HRR or 11–14 RPE. Vigorous: 60%–85% of HRR or ≥15 on Borg scale.	20–60 min.	Dynamic use of large muscle groups.
Strength training	2–3 d per wk.	2–3 sets of 8–12 repetitions. 12–16 RPE.	30 min.	8–10 exercises targeting major muscle groups.
Flexibility	Most days of the week.	Stretch to tightness but not to pain.	15–30 seconds/ stretch. Repeat 2–4 times.	Static stretches targeting major muscle groups.

Abbreviations: FITT, frequency, intensity, time, type; HRR, heart rate reserve; RPE, rate of perceived exertion according to 6–20 Borg scale.

Another principle that is not included in the FITT acronym is exercise progression. Progressions to exercise must be considered when adaptations occur and the patient becomes accustomed to the demands of the exercise performed. This basic training principle is necessary to ensure that the body is continuously stressed, allowing for optimal improvements.[90] Overloading or progressing the exercise program accordingly can be achieved by increasing either one of the FITT variables; however, it is recommended to increase frequency and duration before intensity.[91]

Although there are yet to be specific exercise guidelines for patients awaiting surgery, there is evidence that preoperative exercise improves functional and cardiorespiratory fitness, strength, quality of life, and more. However, it is not clear if this improvement in fitness translates into reduced perioperative risk or improved postoperative outcomes.[92,93]

Role of Nutrition to Increase Muscle Strength

The nutritional status of patients scheduled for surgery is directly influenced by the presence of cancer, which has an impact on all aspects of intermediary metabolism. The primary goal of nutrition therapy is to optimize nutrient stores preoperatively and provide adequate nutrition to compensate for the catabolic response of surgery postoperatively.[94–97] To be successful, a nutrition intervention requires a timeline that needs to start with preoperative assessment and extend into the postoperative period. The greater sensitivity of protein catabolism to nutritional support, in particular to amino acids, could have important implications for the nutritional management of these patients during periods of catabolic stress, with particular emphasis on substrate utilization and energy requirement during the healing process. Protein intake is calculated as 20% of total energy expenditure, determined individually, using a stress factor of 1.3 for major surgery and an appropriate activity factor.[44] Protein requirements are elevated in stressed states, such as cancer, to account for added demands of hepatic acute phase proteins synthesis, and the synthesis of proteins involved in immune function and wound healing. Nonsurgical nutrition oncology guidelines on enteral nutrition suggest that patients with cancer should consume at least 1.2 to 2.0 g protein/kg per day.

Dietary protein increases whole body protein synthesis by increasing systemic amino acid availability. After exercise, the ingestion of amino acids is recommended because of the stimulatory effect that amino acids have on muscle protein synthesis[98,99] (**Fig. 4**). In fact, protein ingestion post resistance exercise has been found to stimulate rates of myofibrillar protein synthesis above fasting rates for 24 hours.[100]

Psychological Distress Before Surgery

The presence of psychological distress, specifically anxiety and depression, is very common in patients with cancer. In fact, Hellstadius and colleagues[101] found that 34% and 23% of patients with esophageal cancer waiting for surgery were considered

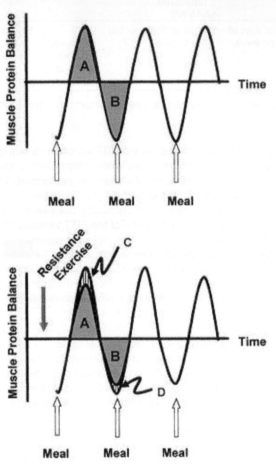

Fig. 4. Top: Normal fed–state protein synthesis and fasted-state protein breakdown. The area under the curve in the fed state (A) is equivalent to the fasted loss area under the curve (B); hence, skeletal muscle mass is maintained by feeding. Bottom: Fed-state protein synthesis and fasted-state protein breakdown in skeletal muscle with performance of resistance exercise. Fasted-state gains are enhanced by an amount equivalent to the stimulation of protein synthesis brought about by exercise (C). Additionally, fasted-state losses appear to be less (D), due to persistent stimulation of protein synthesis in the fasted state. (*Adapted from* Phillips SM. Protein requirements and supplementation in strength sports. Nutrition 2004;20(7):691; with permission.)

anxious and depressed, respectively. Such mental states have shown to negatively impact surgical and clinical outcomes, such as wound healing, postoperative pain relief, hospital stay, and functional recovery even after known physiologic factors were accounted for.[102] There is evidence in breast, colon, and prostate cancer supporting the role of psychological interventions implemented before surgery to alleviate distress, improve quality of life,[103] reduce anxiety and depression,[103,104] and reduce pain severity and fatigue.[105] These interventions include relaxation techniques (deep breathing, progressive muscle relaxation, and meditation), guided imagery, and/or problem-solving and coping strategies. However, these strategies did not affect traditional surgical outcomes, including length of hospital stay, complications, analgesic use, or mortality.[106]

Further Steps

The increasing interest in prehabilitation for surgical cancer patients stems from growing, however limited, evidence that such multidisciplinary programs can address modifiable risk factors that may impact treatment outcomes.[107] Additionally, in the patient perspective, prehabilitation shows promising effects on preoperative functional capacity in anticipation of surgery, and with more research could mitigate the pathophysiological burden associated with cancer and surgical stress, thus accelerating the recovery process. Patients with limited reserve can potentially benefit more from a structured personalized prehabilitation program, as shown recently.[72] Although the prehabilitation approach has the potential for diagnosing reversible limitations in the preoperative period and targeting intervention strategies to ameliorate postoperative outcomes, there are still gaps in our understanding of how to identify those patients who would benefit from the prehabilitation program, select the appropriate interventions, determine the effectiveness in the context of a definite type if surgery, and examine the impact on patient-centered and clinical outcomes. More needs to be done and knowledge to be acquired with respect to the prescription of exercise and the role of immunonutrition within the context of ERAS programs for each specific type of surgery. This patient-centered, multidisciplinary, and integrated medical care program should start in the preoperative clinic where vulnerable patients can be identified, risk stratified adequately by an interdisciplinary team with the aim of improving surgical outcome, and promoting healthy behaviors throughout the continuum of care.

REFERENCES

1. White PF, Kehlet H, Neal JM, et al. The role of the anesthesiologist in fast-track surgery: from multimodal analgesia to perioperative medical care. Anesth Analg 2007;104(6):1380–96 [Table of contents].

2. Kehlet H, Wilmore DW. Evidence-based surgical care and the evolution of fast-track surgery. Ann Surg 2008;248(2):189–98.

3. Fearon KC, Ljungqvist O, Von Meyenfeldt M, et al. Enhanced recovery after surgery: a consensus review of clinical care for patients undergoing colonic resection. Clin Nutr 2005;24(3):466–77.

4. Eskicioglu C, Forbes SS, Aarts MA, et al. Enhanced recovery after surgery (ERAS) programs for patients having colorectal surgery: a meta-analysis of randomized trials. J Gastrointest Surg 2009;13(12):2321–9.

5. Gouvas N, Tan E, Windsor A, et al. Fast-track vs standard care in colorectal surgery: a meta-analysis update. Int J Colorectal Dis 2009;24(10):1119–31.

6. Lassen K, Soop M, Nygren J, et al. Consensus review of optimal perioperative care in colorectal surgery: Enhanced Recovery After Surgery (ERAS) Group recommendations. Arch Surg 2009;144(10):961–9.

7. Kehlet H, Wilmore DW. Surgical care—how can new evidence be applied to clinical practice? Colorectal Dis 2010;12(1):2–4.

8. Wilmore DW. Metabolic response to severe surgical illness: overview. World J Surg 2000;24(6):705–11.

9. Carli F. Physiologic considerations of Enhanced Recovery After Surgery (ERAS) programs: implications of the stress response. Can J Anaesth 2015;62(2):110–9.

10. Baldini G, Fawcett WJ. Anesthesia for colorectal surgery. Anesthesiol Clin 2015;33(1):93–123.

11. Duceppe E, Parlow J, MacDonald P, et al. Canadian cardiovascular society guidelines on perioperative cardiac risk assessment and management for patients who undergo noncardiac surgery. Can J Cardiol 2017;33(1):17–32.

12. Junejo MA, Mason JM, Sheen AJ, et al. Cardiopulmonary exercise testing for preoperative risk assessment before hepatic resection. Br J Surg 2012;99(8):1097–104.

13. Junejo MA, Mason JM, Sheen AJ, et al. Cardiopulmonary exercise testing for preoperative risk assessment before pancreaticoduodenectomy for cancer. Ann Surg Oncol 2014;21(6):1929–36.

14. Lee L, Schwartzman K, Carli F, et al. The association of the distance walked in 6 min with pre-operative peak oxygen consumption and complications 1 month after colorectal resection. Anaesthesia 2013;68(8):811–6.

15. Pecorelli N, Fiore JF Jr, Gillis C, et al. The six-minute walk test as a measure of postoperative recovery after colorectal resection: further examination of its measurement properties. Surg Endosc 2016;30(6):2199–206.

16. Moriello C, Mayo NE, Feldman L, et al. Validating the six-minute walk test as a measure of recovery after elective colon resection surgery. Arch Phys Med Rehabil 2008;89(6):1083–9.

17. Feldheiser A, Aziz O, Baldini G, et al. Enhanced Recovery After Surgery (ERAS) for gastrointestinal surgery, part 2: consensus statement for anaesthesia practice. Acta Anaesthesiol Scand 2016;60(3):289–334.

18. Nyasavajjala SM, Low J. Anaerobic threshold: pitfalls and limitations. Anaesthesia 2009;64(9):934–6.

19. Lim E, Baldwin D, Beckles M, et al. Guidelines on the radical management of patients with lung cancer. Thorax 2010;65(Suppl 3):iii1–27.

20. McCullough PA, Gallagher MJ, Dejong AT, et al. Cardiorespiratory fitness and short-term complications after bariatric surgery. Chest 2006;130(2):517–25.

21. Snowden CP, Prentis JM, Anderson HL, et al. Submaximal cardiopulmonary exercise testing predicts complications and hospital length of stay in patients undergoing major elective surgery. Ann Surg 2010;251(3):535–41.

22. West MA, Lythgoe D, Barben CP, et al. Cardiopulmonary exercise variables are associated with postoperative morbidity after major colonic surgery: a prospective blinded observational study. Br J Anaesth 2014;112(4):665–71.

23. Forshaw MJ, Strauss DC, Davies AR, et al. Is cardiopulmonary exercise testing a useful test before esophagectomy? Ann Thorac Surg 2008;85(1):294–9.

24. Nagamatsu Y, Shima I, Yamana H, et al. Preoperative evaluation of cardiopulmonary reserve with the use of expired gas analysis during exercise testing in patients with squamous cell carcinoma of the thoracic esophagus. J Thorac Cardiovasc Surg 2001;121(6):1064–8.

25. Nugent AM, Riley M, Megarry J, et al. Cardiopulmonary exercise testing in the pre-operative assessment of patients for repair of abdominal aortic aneurysm. Ir J Med Sci 1998;167(4):238–41.
26. Smith TB, Stonell C, Purkayastha S, et al. Cardiopulmonary exercise testing as a risk assessment method in non cardio-pulmonary surgery: a systematic review. Anaesthesia 2009;64(8):883–93.
27. Older P, Smith R, Courtney P, et al. Preoperative evaluation of cardiac failure and ischemia in elderly patients by cardiopulmonary exercise testing. Chest 1993; 104(3):701–4.
28. Older P, Hall A, Hader R. Cardiopulmonary exercise testing as a screening test for perioperative management of major surgery in the elderly. Chest 1999; 116(2):355–62.
29. Wilson RJ, Davies S, Yates D, et al. Impaired functional capacity is associated with all-cause mortality after major elective intra-abdominal surgery. Br J Anaesth 2010;105(3):297–303.
30. Grant SW, Hickey GL, Wisely NA, et al. Cardiopulmonary exercise testing and survival after elective abdominal aortic aneurysm repair. Br J Anaesth 2015; 114(3):430–6.
31. Carlisle J, Swart M. Mid-term survival after abdominal aortic aneurysm surgery predicted by cardiopulmonary exercise testing. Br J Surg 2007;94(8):966–9.
32. Epstein SK, Freeman RB, Khayat A, et al. Aerobic capacity is associated with 100-day outcome after hepatic transplantation. Liver Transpl 2004;10(3): 418–24.
33. Colson M, Baglin J, Bolsin S, et al. Cardiopulmonary exercise testing predicts 5 yr survival after major surgery. Br J Anaesth 2012;109(5):735–41.
34. West MA, Loughney L, Lythgoe D, et al. Effect of prehabilitation on objectively measured physical fitness after neoadjuvant treatment in preoperative rectal cancer patients: a blinded interventional pilot study. Br J Anaesth 2015; 114(2):244–51.
35. Musallam KM, Tamim HM, Richards T, et al. Preoperative anaemia and postoperative outcomes in non-cardiac surgery: a retrospective cohort study. Lancet 2011;378(9800):1396–407.
36. Knight K, Wade S, Balducci L. Prevalence and outcomes of anemia in cancer: a systematic review of the literature. Am J Med 2004;116(Suppl 7A):11S–26S.
37. Cata JP. Perioperative anemia and blood transfusions in patients with cancer: when the problem, the solution, and their combination are each associated with poor outcomes. Anesthesiology 2015;122(1):3–4.
38. Goodnough LT, Shander A. Patient blood management. Anesthesiology 2012; 116(6):1367–76.
39. Hare GM, Baker JE, Pavenski K. Assessment and treatment of preoperative anemia: continuing professional development. Can J Anaesth 2011;58(6): 569–81.
40. Shander A, Javidroozi M, Ozawa S, et al. What is really dangerous: anaemia or transfusion? Br J Anaesth 2011;107(Suppl 1):i41–59.
41. Hallet J, Hanif A, Callum J, et al. The impact of perioperative iron on the use of red blood cell transfusions in gastrointestinal surgery: a systematic review and meta-analysis. Transfus Med Rev 2014;28(4):205–11.
42. Meybohm P, Herrmann E, Steinbicker AU, et al. Patient blood management is associated with a substantial reduction of red blood cell utilization and safe for patient's outcome: a prospective, multicenter cohort study with a noninferiority design. Ann Surg 2016;264(2):203–11.

43. Huhmann MB, August DA. Perioperative nutrition support in cancer patients. Nutr Clin Pract 2012;27(5):586–92.
44. Weimann A, Braga M, Carli F, et al. ESPEN guideline: clinical nutrition in surgery. Clin Nutr 2017;36(3):623–50.
45. Gupta D, Lis CG. Pretreatment serum albumin as a predictor of cancer survival: a systematic review of the epidemiological literature. Nutr J 2010;9:69.
46. Arends J, Baracos V, Bertz H, et al. ESPEN expert group recommendations for action against cancer-related malnutrition. Clin Nutr 2017;36(5):1187–96.
47. Kabata P, Jastrzebski T, Kakol M, et al. Preoperative nutritional support in cancer patients with no clinical signs of malnutrition—prospective randomized controlled trial. Support Care Cancer 2015;23(2):365–70.
48. Jie B, Jiang ZM, Nolan MT, et al. Impact of preoperative nutritional support on clinical outcome in abdominal surgical patients at nutritional risk. Nutrition 2012;28(10):1022–7.
49. Buijs N, van Bokhorst-de van der Schueren MA, Langius JA, et al. Perioperative arginine-supplemented nutrition in malnourished patients with head and neck cancer improves long-term survival. Am J Clin Nutr 2010;92(5):1151–6.
50. Gustafsson UO, Oppelstrup H, Thorell A, et al. Adherence to the ERAS protocol is associated with 5-year survival after colorectal cancer surgery: a retrospective cohort study. World J Surg 2016;40(7):1741–7.
51. Horowitz M, Neeman E, Sharon E, et al. Exploiting the critical perioperative period to improve long-term cancer outcomes. Nat Rev Clin Oncol 2015; 12(4):213–26.
52. Thomsen T, Villebro N, Moller AM. Interventions for preoperative smoking cessation. Cochrane Database Syst Rev 2014;3:CD002294.
53. Wong J, Abrishami A, Yang Y, et al. A perioperative smoking cessation intervention with varenicline: a double-blind, randomized, placebo-controlled trial. Anesthesiology 2012;117(4):755–64.
54. Ip HY, Abrishami A, Peng PW, et al. Predictors of postoperative pain and analgesic consumption: a qualitative systematic review. Anesthesiology 2009; 111(3):657–77.
55. Chow WB, Rosenthal RA, Merkow RP, et al. Optimal preoperative assessment of the geriatric surgical patient: a best practices guideline from the American College of Surgeons National Surgical Quality Improvement Program and the American Geriatrics Society. J Am Coll Surg 2012;215(4):453–66.
56. Blitz JD, Kendale SM, Jain SK, et al. Preoperative evaluation clinic visit is associated with decreased risk of in-hospital postoperative mortality. Anesthesiology 2016;125(2):280–94.
57. Fleisher LA, Fleischmann KE, Auerbach AD, et al. 2014 ACC/AHA guideline on perioperative cardiovascular evaluation and management of patients undergoing noncardiac surgery: executive summary: a report of the American College of Cardiology/American Heart Association Task Force on practice guidelines. Developed in collaboration with the American College of Surgeons, American Society of Anesthesiologists, American Society of Echocardiography, American Society of Nuclear Cardiology, Heart Rhythm Society, Society for Cardiovascular Angiography and Interventions, Society of Cardiovascular Anesthesiologists, and Society of Vascular Medicine Endorsed by the Society of Hospital Medicine. J Nucl Cardiol 2015;22(1):162–215.
58. Qaseem A, Snow V, Fitterman N, et al. Risk assessment for and strategies to reduce perioperative pulmonary complications for patients undergoing

noncardiothoracic surgery: a guideline from the American College of Physicians. Ann Intern Med 2006;144(8):575–80.

59. Ebert TJ, Shankar H, Haake RM. Perioperative considerations for patients with morbid obesity. Anesthesiol Clin 2006;24(3):621–36.

60. American Society of Anesthesiologists Task Force on Perioperative Management of patients with obstructive sleep apnea. Practice guidelines for the perioperative management of patients with obstructive sleep apnea: an updated report by the American Society of Anesthesiologists Task Force on Perioperative Management of patients with obstructive sleep apnea. Anesthesiology 2014; 120(2):268–86.

61. Moghissi ES, Korytkowski MT, DiNardo M, et al. American Association of Clinical Endocrinologists and American Diabetes Association consensus statement on inpatient glycemic control. Diabetes Care 2009;32(6):1119–31.

62. Sahai SK, Zalpour A, Rozner MA. Preoperative evaluation of the oncology patient. Med Clin North Am 2010;94(2):403–19.

63. Pearse RM, Harrison DA, James P, et al. Identification and characterisation of the high-risk surgical population in the United Kingdom. Crit Care 2006; 10(3):R81.

64. Fearon KC, Jenkins JT, Carli F, et al. Patient optimization for gastrointestinal cancer surgery. Br J Surg 2013;100(1):15–27.

65. Older P, Smith R, Hall A, et al. Preoperative cardiopulmonary risk assessment by cardiopulmonary exercise testing. Crit Care Resusc 2000;2(3):198–208.

66. Ditmyer MM, Topp R, Pifer M. Prehabilitation in preparation for orthopaedic surgery. Orthop Nurs 2002;21(5):43–51 [quiz: 52–4].

67. Topp R, Ditmyer M, King K, et al. The effect of bed rest and potential of prehabilitation on patients in the intensive care unit. AACN Clin Issues 2002;13(2): 263–76.

68. Valkenet K, van de Port IG, Dronkers JJ, et al. The effects of preoperative exercise therapy on postoperative outcome: a systematic review. Clin Rehabil 2011; 25(2):99–111.

69. Santa Mina D, Clarke H, Ritvo P, et al. Effect of total-body prehabilitation on postoperative outcomes: a systematic review and meta-analysis. Physiotherapy 2014;100(3):196–207.

70. Lemanu DP, Singh PP, MacCormick AD, et al. Effect of preoperative exercise on cardiorespiratory function and recovery after surgery: a systematic review. World J Surg 2013;37(4):711–20.

71. Carli F, Charlebois P, Stein B, et al. Randomized clinical trial of prehabilitation in colorectal surgery. Br J Surg 2010;97(8):1187–97.

72. Minnella EM, Bousquet-Dion G, Awasthi R, et al. Multimodal prehabilitation improves functional capacity before and after colorectal surgery for cancer: a five-year research experience. Acta Oncol 2017;56(2):295–300.

73. Li C, Carli F, Lee L, et al. Impact of a trimodal prehabilitation program on functional recovery after colorectal cancer surgery: a pilot study. Surg Endosc 2013; 27(4):1072–82.

74. Gillis C, Li C, Lee L, et al. Prehabilitation versus rehabilitation: a randomized control trial in patients undergoing colorectal resection for cancer. Anesthesiology 2014;121(5):937–47.

75. Mujika I, Padilla S. Cardiorespiratory and metabolic characteristics of detraining in humans. Med Sci Sports Exerc 2001;33(3):413–21.

76. Bienso RS, Ringholm S, Kiilerich K, et al. GLUT4 and glycogen synthase are key players in bed rest-induced insulin resistance. Diabetes 2012;61(5):1090–9.

77. Sonne MP, Hojbjerre L, Alibegovic AC, et al. Endothelial function after 10 days of bed rest in individuals at risk for type 2 diabetes and cardiovascular disease. Exp Physiol 2011;96(10):1000–9.

78. Minnella EM, Awasthi R, Gillis C, et al. Patients with poor baseline walking capacity are most likely to improve their functional status with multimodal prehabilitation. Surgery 2016;160(4):1070–9.

79. Ferreira V, Agnihotram RV, Bergdahl A, et al. Maximizing patient adherence to prehabilitation: what do the patients say? Support Care Cancer 2018;26(8): 2717–23.

80. Nelson ME, Rejeski WJ, Blair SN, et al. Physical activity and public health in older adults: recommendation from the American College of Sports Medicine and the American Heart Association. Med Sci Sports Exerc 2007;39(8): 1435–45.

81. O'Doherty AF, West M, Jack S, et al. Preoperative aerobic exercise training in elective intra-cavity surgery: a systematic review. Br J Anaesth 2013;110(5): 679–89.

82. Speck RM, Courneya KS, Masse LC, et al. An update of controlled physical activity trials in cancer survivors: a systematic review and meta-analysis. J Cancer Surviv 2010;4(2):87–100.

83. Schmidt K, Vogt L, Thiel C, et al. Validity of the six-minute walk test in cancer patients. Int J Sports Med 2013;34(7):631–6.

84. Fielding RA. The role of progressive resistance training and nutrition in the preservation of lean body mass in the elderly. J Am Coll Nutr 1995;14(6):587–94.

85. Watters JM, Clancey SM, Moulton SB, et al. Impaired recovery of strength in older patients after major abdominal surgery. Ann Surg 1993;218(3):380–90 [discussion: 390–3].

86. Rikli RE, Jones CJ. Development and validation of criterion-referenced clinically relevant fitness standards for maintaining physical independence in later years. Gerontologist 2013;53(2):255–67.

87. Kenney WL, Humphrey RH, Bryant CX, et al. ACSM's guidelines for exercise testing and prescription. 5th edition. Baltimore (MD): Williams & Wilkins; 1995.

88. Borg G. Perceived exertion as an indicator of somatic stress. Scand J Rehabil Med 1970;2(2):92–8.

89. Borg GA. Psychophysical bases of perceived exertion. Med Sci Sports Exerc 1982;14(5):377–81.

90. McDermott AY, Mernitz H. Exercise and older patients: prescribing guidelines. Am Fam Physician 2006;74(3):437–44.

91. Rajarajeswaran P, Vishnupriya R. Exercise in cancer. Indian J Med Paediatr Oncol 2009;30(2):61–70.

92. Boereboom C, Doleman B, Lund JN, et al. Systematic review of pre-operative exercise in colorectal cancer patients. Tech Coloproctol 2016;20(2):81–9.

93. Pouwels S, Stokmans RA, Willigendael EM, et al. Preoperative exercise therapy for elective major abdominal surgery: a systematic review. Int J Surg 2014;12(2): 134–40.

94. Schwegler I, von Holzen A, Gutzwiller JP, et al. Nutritional risk is a clinical predictor of postoperative mortality and morbidity in surgery for colorectal cancer. Br J Surg 2010;97(1):92–7.

95. Howard L, Ashley C. Nutrition in the perioperative patient. Annu Rev Nutr 2003; 23:263–82.

96. Weimann A, Braga M, Harsanyi L, et al. ESPEN guidelines on enteral nutrition: surgery including organ transplantation. Clin Nutr 2006;25(2):224–44.

97. McClave SA, Kozar R, Martindale RG, et al. Summary points and consensus recommendations from the North American Surgical Nutrition Summit. JPEN J Parenter Enteral Nutr 2013;37(5 Suppl):99S–105S.
98. Esmarck B, Andersen JL, Olsen S, et al. Timing of postexercise protein intake is important for muscle hypertrophy with resistance training in elderly humans. J Physiol 2001;535(Pt 1):301–11.
99. Burke LM, Hawley JA, Ross ML, et al. Preexercise aminoacidemia and muscle protein synthesis after resistance exercise. Med Sci Sports Exerc 2012;44(10): 1968–77.
100. Biolo G, Tipton KD, Klein S, et al. An abundant supply of amino acids enhances the metabolic effect of exercise on muscle protein. Am J Physiol 1997;273(1 Pt 1):E122–9.
101. Hellstadius Y, Lagergren J, Zylstra J, et al. Prevalence and predictors of anxiety and depression among esophageal cancer patients prior to surgery. Dis Esophagus 2016;29(8):1128–34.
102. Rosenberger PH, Jokl P, Ickovics J. Psychosocial factors and surgical outcomes: an evidence-based literature review. J Am Acad Orthop Surg 2006; 14(7):397–405.
103. Garssen B, Boomsma MF, Meezenbroek Ede J, et al. Stress management training for breast cancer surgery patients. Psychooncology 2013;22(3):572–80.
104. Parker PA, Pettaway CA, Babaian RJ, et al. The effects of a presurgical stress management intervention for men with prostate cancer undergoing radical prostatectomy. J Clin Oncol 2009;27(19):3169–76.
105. Larson MR, Duberstein PR, Talbot NL, et al. A presurgical psychosocial intervention for breast cancer patients. psychological distress and the immune response. J Psychosom Res 2000;48(2):187–94.
106. Tsimopoulou I, Pasquali S, Howard R, et al. Psychological prehabilitation before cancer surgery: a systematic review. Ann Surg Oncol 2015;22(13):4117–23.
107. Silver JK, Baima J, Mayer RS. Impairment-driven cancer rehabilitation: an essential component of quality care and survivorship. CA Cancer J Clin 2013; 63(5):295–317.

Enhanced Recovery After Surgery and Multimodal Strategies for Analgesia

W. Jonathan Dunkman, MD*, Michael W. Manning, MD, PhD

KEYWORDS

- Enhanced recovery after surgery • Multimodal analgesia • Nonopioid analgesics
- Regional anesthesia

KEY POINTS

- Enhanced recovery after surgery is an evidenced-based, multidisciplinary, multimodal approach to patient care during the perioperative period, of which a comprehensive analgesic plan is critical to overall success.
- Opioids have been the foundation of all analgesic strategies for more than 100 years but carry significant risks and side effects including morbidity and mortality.
- Careful attention to analgesia choices through selection of nonopioid, multimodal approaches including regional techniques, can permit the significant reduction of or elimination of opioids.

INTRODUCTION

Enhanced recovery after surgery (ERAS) is an evidence-based, multidisciplinary, multimodal approach to the perioperative care of a patient undergoing surgery. Enhanced recovery pathways seek to attenuate the stress response to surgery and maintain endocrine and metabolic homeostasis facilitating postoperative recovery. A variety of interventions throughout the preoperative, intraoperative and postoperative periods are designed to modulate the neurohormonal response to surgery, minimizing the deleterious effects, such as catabolism, increased cardiac demands, and exaggerated inflammatory responses, while preserving the beneficial effects, such as immune function and wound healing.[1,2]

Analgesia is a critical component of an enhanced recovery pathway. Local or regional anesthetics and systemic analgesics block or attenuate the nociceptive inputs that feed the stress response to surgery. Optimal pain relief is also critical for patients to mobilize quickly after surgery, a critical component of enhanced recovery with

Disclosure Statement: The authors have nothing to disclose.
Department of Anesthesiology, Duke University, Duke University Medical Center, Box 3094, Durham, NC 27710, USA
* Corresponding author.
E-mail address: william.dunkman@duke.edu

downstream effects in terms of preventing complications, such as infection and thromboembolism. Pain control with a manageable analgesic regimen is also critical to achieving recovery milestones and preparing for discharge. In selecting an analgesic regimen for enhanced recovery, care must be taken to avoid the negative side effects of analgesic treatments that may impair recovery or predispose to complications.[3,4]

Traditional analgesic regimens for major surgery relied heavily on opioids, which do provide analgesia, but which can cause to a wide range of serious side effects, including postoperative nausea and vomiting (PONV), constipation, ileus, sedation, respiratory depression, and urinary retention, which can impair and not enhance a patient's recovery. Enhanced recovery protocols should therefore incorporate multimodal analgesic strategies that minimize opioid use and optimize analgesia while minimizing side effects. These modalities may include neuraxial or regional anesthesia, local anesthesia, long-acting local anesthetics, acetaminophen, nonsteroidal anti-inflammatory drugs (NSAIDs), gabapentenoids, N-methyl-D-aspartate (NMDA) receptor antagonists, systemic lidocaine, α_2-agonists, and glucocorticoids, among other options.[4,5] A recent review of enhanced recovery protocols for major abdomino-pelvic surgery found that neuraxial/regional anesthesia, acetaminophen, and NSAIDs are used most commonly.[5]

The initial concept of enhanced recovery and the earliest full-fledged enhanced recovery pathways focused only on colorectal surgery. By far, most of the literature and data on enhanced recovery focuses on major abdominal surgery generally and on colorectal surgery in particular. As such, this review can be read as specifically applying to major abdominal surgery, although many of the principles can be extrapolated to other forms of surgery.

For example, regional anesthesia strategies are used with great success in orthopedic and breast surgery and can provide the base for multimodal analgesia for these types of surgeries. Many of the nonopioid pain analgesics discussed here could be used for a variety of surgeries. A similar strategy of opioid minimization is valuable in a variety of situations. Thoughtful application of these principles can lead to a valuable multimodal analgesic plan across the surgical spectrum.

FRAMEWORK FOR MULTIMODAL ANALGESIA

Multimodal analgesia is thought of in several steps or layers, with elements from each layer chosen based on the specific patient and surgery (**Fig. 1**). The first layer in any analgesic plan should be regional or local anesthesia tailored to the invasiveness of the operation. This may be chosen on a spectrum from a thoracic epidural for a major open operation or spinal analgesia or truncal blocks for laparoscopic surgery through local infiltration for a small procedure. The next step is nonopioid systemic analgesics. This lays a strong foundation for analgesia and modulating the stress response, ideally with drugs from several different therapeutic categories, with thought to side effects and patient comorbidities in selecting various drugs. Systemic opioids can then be used sparingly as a rescue medication or to cover areas of inadequate block coverage.

REGIONAL AND LOCAL ANESTHESIA
Epidural Analgesia

Thoracic epidural analgesia (TEA) remains the gold standard for regional anesthesia in major abdominal surgery, having been shown to provide superior analgesia versus parental opioids.[6,7] TEA shows clear benefits and has long been accepted as the analgesic strategy of choice for open abdominal procedures with benefits in length of stay,

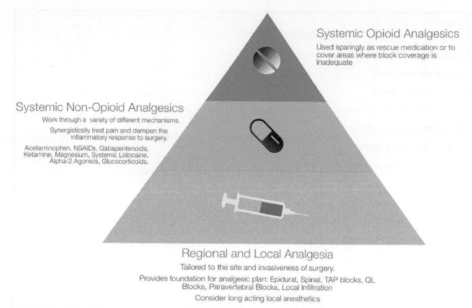

Fig. 1. Multimodal approach to analgesia. QL, quadratus lumborum; TAP, transversus abdominis plane.

morbidity, and mortality. It has also been associated with improvements in mortality and in major cardiopulmonary complications including deep vein thrombosis, pulmonary embolism, transfusion, pneumonia, respiratory depression, myocardial infarction, renal failure, atrial fibrillation, supraventricular tachycardia, and atelectasis.[8,9] TEA also decreases the risk of gastrointestinal complications of particular relevance to enhanced recovery, such as ileus and PONV, which makes it highly desirable especially in gastrointestinal surgery.

TEA is not without risk, however. The same meta-analysis that showed many of these benefits also showed an increased risk arterial hypotension, pruritis, urinary retention, motor blockade, and technical failures, which occurred in 6.1% of patients. Among the rare but potentially serious complications are epidural hematoma, abscess, and neurologic injury.[9]

Despite this, TEA does minimize opioid use and associated negative side effects. A multimodal infusion containing local anesthetic and opioid is common and provides excellent analgesia, although local anesthetic or opioid alone is used in certain patients.[4,10,11] The consensus, in clinical practice and the literature, is that the benefits of TEA substantially outweigh the risks for large open procedures (**Box 1**).

Unfortunately, these benefits are less clear for laparoscopic procedures, and the risks may outweigh the benefits. As advances in minimally invasive surgery and enhanced recovery techniques shorten length of stay and reduce complications, there may be less benefit to epidural analgesia.[12] Recent studies looking specifically at enhanced recovery patients and patients receiving laparoscopic surgery have shown less benefit to epidurals than previous studies.[13,14] TEA may delay early mobilization and even discharge.[15] It is clearly not helpful for a patient to recover quickly from their surgery and remain in the hospital for epidural management. There are other techniques that may provide excellent analgesia and opioid avoidance for laparoscopic procedures without the risks and complications of TEA.[16]

Box 1
Benefits and risks of thoracic epidural analgesia

Benefits of Thoracic Epidural Analgesia

Superior analgesia

Reduced mortality

Reduction in deep venous thromboembolism/pulmonary embolism

Reduction in transfusion

Reduction in pneumonia

Reduction in respiratory depression

Reduction in myocardial infarction

Reduction in renal failure

Reduction in atrial fibrillation

Reduction in supraventricular tachycardia

Reduction in atelectasis

Decreased ileus

Decreased postoperative nausea and vomiting

Risks of Thoracic Epidural Analgesia

Arterial hypotension

Pruritus

Urinary retention

Motor blockade

Technical failures

Epidural hematoma

Epidural abscess

Neurologic injury

As surgery moves to less invasive techniques and enhanced recovery principles speed postoperative recovery, the benefits of epidurals may no longer outweigh the risks and newer analgesic techniques have been developed to fill the gap. Spinal or truncal nerve blocks may offer excellent analgesia for these less invasive surgical techniques with fewer downsides than epidural analgesia.[17]

Spinal Analgesia

Spinal analgesia is emerging as an attractive alternative for laparoscopic procedures within an enhanced recovery pathway. Intrathecal opioid alone (without local anesthetic) has been shown to decrease pain following abdominal surgery.[18] Several groups have shown good results with intrathecal opioid and local anesthetic placed preoperatively in conjunction with a general anesthetic. In comparison with a sham procedure and intravenous (IV) opioid, it decreased length of stay, postoperative pain, and postoperative opioid use.[19] In a study comparing epidural, spinal, and opioid patient-controlled analgesia (PCA) analgesics, spinal and PCA techniques showed shorter length of stay and return of bowel function than epidural analgesia for laparoscopic colorectal surgery within an enhanced recovery protocol. Spinal analgesia had improved postoperative pain versus PCA.[20]

Multimodal low-dose spinals with a low dose of local anesthetic and a low dose of opioid result in faster recovery of sensory and motor function and lower the risk of hypotension compared with traditional dosing.[4,21] The intrathecal opioid is probably responsible for most of the postoperative analgesia associated with this technique, with the expected duration of action in the 24- to 48-hour range. The local anesthetic is helpful for providing dense analgesia in the operative and immediately postoperative period, with duration of action expected in the 6- to 8-hour range. This dense block at the time of surgical insult may also provide additional downstream benefits by partially blocking the stress response associated with these operations.[22]

Spinal analgesia is a safe and well-established technique but it is not without complications or safety concerns of which pruritus and PONV are some of the most common. Intrathecal opioids have also been associated with delayed respiratory depression and caution must be used, particularly if additional opioids or other sedative medications are given in the postoperative period. Additional monitoring or close supervision within an institutional plan for additional analgesics within the enhanced recovery pathway may be helpful.[19] Many of the procedure-related complications, such as bleeding, trauma, or infection, are similar to those seen with TEA but are rare and probably less common than with TEA because of the smaller needle and lack of introduction of a catheter.

Transversus Abdominis Plane Blocks

Truncal blocks, such as the transversus abdominis plane (TAP) block, offer analgesic options somewhere between neuraxial techniques and local infiltration in terms of invasiveness and efficacy. The TAP block involves injection of local anesthetic into the neurovascular plane between the internal oblique and transversus abdominis muscles via the lumbar triangles of Petit to block the afferent nerves of the abdominal wall. This procedure may be expected to block nerves in the T7 to L1 dermatomes,[23] although coverage seems to be best below the umbilicus. A subcostal approach may offer better analgesia at higher dermatomes.[24] This block was initially described using a landmark-based "double-pop" technique[25] but is now commonly performed using ultrasound guidance.[17,26]

TAP blocks are effective at blocking somatic pain from a surgical incision but are not designed or expected to block visceral or sympathetically mediated pain. They have been shown to reduce pain and opioid use postoperatively[25,27] but were not as effective as TEA for radical gastrectomy.[28] Results compared with local infiltration have been mixed but generally positive.[28–31] TAP blocks are generally safe and may be an option in patients for whom neuraxial anesthesia is not possible. The role of TAP blocks in enhanced recovery protocols is still evolving. They may offer a valuable way to deliver regional anesthesia as part of a multimodal analgesic strategy for less invasive surgical procedures.[4,17,32]

Quadratus Lumborum Blocks

Quadratus lumborum blocks are a form of truncal block somewhat similar to TAP blocks but more proximal. They are placed under ultrasound guidance by one of several techniques. They have been shown to more reliably block the T8-10 dermatomes compared with TAP blocks. The precise technique and role of these blocks is still evolving but they may offer a valuable analgesic option in the future.[32,33]

Paravertebral Blocks

Paravertebral nerve blocks (PVB) is a well-established technique for analgesia following thoracotomy, as either a single shot block or as a continuous infusion catheter.[34] It has also been used successfully following outpatient surgeries, such as inguinal herniorrhaphy[35] and breast surgery.[36] PVB can provide analgesia at different levels depending where the block is placed. PVB use is associated with faster recovery times, shorter length of stay, and good pain control, all important goals within an enhanced recovery paradigm.[4] A recent review of PVB for abdominal surgery found generally improved pain scores and decreased opioid requirements but insufficient evidence to draw definitive conclusions compared with other techniques.[37] PVB is a good option to consider alongside other truncal nerve blocks for appropriate procedures.

Local Infiltration

Surgical site infiltration with local anesthetic is an appropriate part of multimodal analgesia when other types of regional analgesia are not necessary or possible. This may entail intraperitoneal local anesthetic, port site infiltration, or other infiltration of the surgical field or incision. A recent review found a statistically significant benefit for intraperitoneal local anesthetic in reducing pain scores and opioid use, but the effect size is of questionable clinical significance. They did not find sufficient evidence to support port site infiltration.[38] One should expect only modest results from local infiltration but it may be reasonable for smaller surgeries where neuraxial or regional techniques are not needed or for larger surgeries where these techniques might be desirable but are contraindicated.

Long-Acting Local Anesthetics

Prolonged pain relief following surgery is usually desirable and local and regional techniques have traditionally favored the longer acting local anesthetics, such as bupivacaine or ropivacaine. More recently, liposomal bupivacaine has become available. This encapsulated formulation of bupivacaine is released over several days as multivesicular liposomes are metabolized by normal biologic processes. Bupivacaine liposome injectable suspension (Exparel) is used for surgical site infiltration and field blocks, such as TAP blocks.[39] TAP blocks with liposomal bupivacaine have been shown to reduce pain scores and opioid use for 24 to 36 hours following colorectal surgery.[40] Long-acting local anesthetics, such as liposomal bupivacaine, may enhance the duration of local and regional analgesic techniques.

SYSTEMIC NONOPIOID ANALGESICS

The next layer of multimodal analgesia is systemic nonopioid analgesics. These work through a variety of mechanisms and synergistically treat pain and dampen the inflammatory response to surgery. They require some thought to side effects in particular patients but are generally well tolerated. A thoughtful selection of several nonopioid analgesics working by different mechanisms should be a part of any enhanced recovery pathway.

Acetaminophen

Acetaminophen is an effective analgesic for mild to moderate pain and is associated with a decrease in pain and opioid usage as part of a multimodal regimen for surgery. It is given orally, IV, or rectally. Oral acetaminophen is cheap and effective and is given preoperatively or postoperatively once oral intake is tolerated. IV acetaminophen is more expensive but is given when a patient is unable to take orally and has favorable pharmacokinetics (faster and more reliable plasma and cerebrospinal fluid concentrations) compared with oral. Rectal acetaminophen has variable absorption and therefore variable analgesic efficacy but is an effective option in certain circumstances.[4,41,42]

Recent meta-analyses of randomized controlled trials have shown that acetaminophen reduces pain at rest, pain with movement, postoperative opioid consumption, and PONV.[43,44] Acetaminophen is generally safe in doses up to 3 to 4 g per day, although lower doses or avoidance may be considered in patients with liver disease.

Nonsteroidal Anti-inflammatory Drugs

NSAIDs are effective analgesic and anti-inflammatory drugs that inhibit cyclooxyge-nase (COX) thereby reducing prostaglandin synthesis. NSAIDs are either nonselective (eg, ibuprofen or ketorolac), meaning they inhibit COX-1 and COX-2, or selective COX-2 inhibitors (eg, celecoxib). COX-2 is the enzyme induced by pain and inflammation and COX-1 is involved with gastrointestinal and platelet function.[22] Both groups are effective analgesics with a mass of studies showing decreased pain and opioid usage as part of a multimodal regimen.[45–51] There are, however, some significant safety concerns with NSAIDs. They can cause platelet dysfunction and prolong bleeding times and as such, nonselective NSAIDs in particular are often withheld. However, a recent meta-analysis found that ketorolac did not increase bleeding[52] and COX-2 inhibitors have minimal effect on bleeding even at high doses.[53] There is also concern that NSAIDs, particularly nonselective NSAIDs, may increase the risk for an anastomotic leak.[54–58] The data are somewhat mixed and of low quality. As such, it is not considered sufficient to recommend against the use of NSAIDs, especially COX-2 specific NSAIDs, at this time given their other significant benefits. Caution may be warranted in patients at risk for bleeding or anastomotic leak, but NSAIDs are a valuable and recommended component of multimodal analgesic regimens.[4,41,42]

γ-Aminobutyric Acid Analogues (Gabapentenoids)

Originally developed as anticonvulsants, gabapentenoids have analgesic properties mediated by the α_2-delta subunits of presynaptic calcium channels and decreased excitatory neurotransmitter release. They are now commonly used in the treatment of chronic neuropathic pain and are also useful perioperatively. The two commonly available drugs are gabapentin and pregabalin. Both have been shown to reduce pain scores and opioid use in meta-analyses.[59,60] They are a valuable addition to a multimodal analgesic regimen but caution must be used with regard to side effects, particularly sedation, dizziness, and visual disturbances.[41,42]

N-Methyl-D-Aspartate Receptor Antagonists

NMDA receptor antagonists, such as ketamine, dextromethorphan, and magnesium, are used perioperatively to improve pain and reduce opioid use and related side effects.[42] Ketamine is administered intravenously in subanesthetic doses as either a bolus or as an intraoperative or postoperative infusion.[41] It has been shown to reduce pain scores and opioid use. Valuably, it is not a respiratory depressant, although it does have dose-dependent side effects of hallucinations, vivid dreams, tachycardia, hypertension, dizziness, and blurred vision.[61] It may be of particular use in patients with chronic pain or chronic opioid use, because NMDA receptors are involved in chronic pain development.[62]

Systemic magnesium also exerts an analgesic effect by antagonism of NMDA receptors. It is typically given intraoperatively as an IV bolus and/or infusion. It has been shown to reduce pain at rest, pain with movement, and opioid use[63] although results have been mixed.[64] None of the studies in a systematic review reported clinical toxicity related to toxic serum levels of magnesium,[63] although respiratory muscle weakness and potentiation of nondepolarizing neuromuscular blockade in particular is a concern that requires careful monitoring.

Systemic Lidocaine

Systemic (IV) lidocaine has analgesic, anti-inflammatory, and antihyperalgesic effects. A meta-analysis studying the effects of perioperative lidocaine infusion found that it was associated with lower pain scores, reduced opioid use, and faster recovery after abdominal surgery. They conclude that perioperative systemic lidocaine is a useful adjunct for pain management. The most common regimen was a preoperative bolus followed by continuous infusion.[65] Lidocaine infusion is a useful adjunct in patients where other local anesthetic approaches, such as regional anesthesia, are not possible. Caution should be used in patients receiving α-agonists or β-blockers.[41]

α_2-Agonists

α_2-Agonists have several properties that are desirable as a perioperative adjunct medication including sedation, hypnosis, anxiolysis, sympatholysis, and analgesia. The commonly used agents are clonidine and dexmedetomidine. A meta-analysis found that both agents decreased pain intensity, postoperative opioid use, and nausea. Clonidine was associated with an increased risk of hypotension and dexmedetomidine was associated with an increased risk of bradycardia.[66] However, a Cochrane review of dexmedetomidine found that it decreased opioid use but did not reduce pain scores and that it was associated with hypotension.[67] α_2-Agonists seem to have mild analgesics effects and are considered as part of a multimodal regimen but their hemodynamic effects should be considered.[41]

Glucocorticoids

Glucocorticoids are used to reduce inflammation in a variety of conditions. They also have well established antiemetic properties and dexamethasone is commonly used as prophylaxis for PONV. There has been increasing work looking at their analgesic properties and although results have been mixed, a recent meta-analysis found a small but statistically significant effect in lowering pain scores and opioid use after surgery. They found no increase in infection or delayed wound healing, although they did find higher blood glucose levels at 24 hours in those patients who received dexamethasone. The long-term effects of perioperative glucocorticoid use are not clear.[68]

SYSTEMIC OPIOID ANALGESICS

Opioids

Opioid minimization is one of the primary tenets of the enhanced recovery pathway. Although opioids do provide excellent analgesia in the short term, they come with a host of undesirable side effects including PONV, urinary retention, constipation, ileus, pruritus, sedation, and respiratory depression (**Box 2**). These side effects can substantially delay a patient's recovery from surgery and may be more unpleasant than the pain they are treating, and so other analgesic methods are preferred. However, once regional/local techniques and nonopioid systemic analgesics have been used, opioids do retain some role for breakthrough pain or inadequate block coverage.[4,5,12,41]

Patients with Chronic Opioid Use

Although minimizing opioids is important in all enhanced recovery patients, avoiding opioids entirely is neither possible nor desirable in patients who take a significant dose of opioids on a chronic basis. These patients are likely to have a physiologic dependence on these medications and may experience withdrawal if they are abruptly stopped or reduced in the perioperative period. These patients should have their baseline opioid requirements continued throughout the perioperative period. They are also

| Box 2 |
Undesirable side effects of opioid analgesics
Postoperative nausea and vomiting
Urinary retention
Constipation
Ileus
Pruritis
Sedation
Respiratory depression

likely to have developed tachyphylaxis or tolerance to these medications and will not respond as well as opioid-naive patients when these drugs are used for acute perioperative pain. If opioids are needed for breakthrough pain, they are likely to require higher doses than opioid-naive patients. All of the multimodal therapies described here are likely to be helpful, minimizing their reliance on opioids for perioperative pain relief. Perioperative pain management is likely to be improved by weaning their opioid medications under the guidance of a pain specialist in the weeks before surgery.

Alvimopam

When systemic opioids are used, peripheral opioid antagonists, such as alvimopam, should be considered. Alvimopam competitively binds mu-receptors in the gastrointestinal tract but has a low blood-brain barrier permeability, limiting its effect at the opioids analgesic site.[5] Alvimopam has been shown to reduce time to gastrointestinal recovery as measured by tolerance of solid food and return of bowel movements and time to discharge after major abdominal surgery.[69,70]

NONPHARMACOLOGIC TECHNIQUES

There are a variety of nonpharmacologic analgesic techniques available, including acupuncture, aromatherapy, music therapy, transcutaneous electrical nerve stimulation, hypnosis, and biofeedback. In general, the efficacy of these techniques is still unproven but there are some studies that suggest they may reduce postoperative pain and total analgesic requirements and corresponding side effects. The risk of most of these therapies is minimal and, if available, they are considered for appropriate patients.[4,42]

SUMMARY

ERAS pathways have improved patient care in the last decade through evidence-based, multidisciplinary, multimodal care pathways designed to speed and enhance a patient's recovery after surgery. A thoughtful approach to analgesia is critical for the success of these pathways. These techniques block or attenuate the stress response to surgery. Analgesia is critical for patients to mobilize after surgery and meet recovery milestones. At the same time, one must choose a regimen that minimizes side effects that may compromise patients' return to normal function. Although the establishment of local pathways is critical to success with ERAS programs, the thoughtful application of these principles can allow for a range of ERAS pathways that are suited to specific institutions and categories of procedures. These pathways may then require thoughtful modification to address individual patients' unique circumstances and comorbidities. A layered multimodal approach involving regional anesthetic techniques, systemic nonopioid analgesics, and limited use of systemic opioid analgesics offers excellent pain control with minimal side effects, enhancing patient recovery, and satisfaction.

REFERENCES

1. Kehlet H, Wilmore DW. Evidence-based surgical care and the evolution of fast-track surgery. Ann Surg 2008;248(2):189–98.
2. Ljungqvist O, Scott M, Fearon KC. Enhanced recovery after surgery: a review. JAMA Surg 2017;152(3):292–8.
3. Helander EM, Billeaud CB, Kline RJ, et al. Multimodal approaches to analgesia in enhanced recovery after surgery pathways. Int Anesthesiol Clin 2017;55(4): 51–69.
4. Tan M, Law LS-C, Gan TJ. Optimizing pain management to facilitate enhanced recovery after surgery pathways. Can J Anaesth 2015;62(2):203–18.
5. Law LS, Lo EA, Gan TJ. Preoperative antiemetic and analgesic management. In: Gan TJ, Thacker JK, Miller TE, et al, editors. Enhanced recovery for major abdominopelvic surgery. American Society for Enhanced Recovery. West Islep (NY): Professional Communications, Inc; 2016. p. 105–20.
6. Block BM, Liu SS, Rowlingson AJ, et al. Efficacy of postoperative epidural analgesia: a meta-analysis. JAMA 2003;290(18):2455–63.
7. Pöpping D, Zahn P, Van Aken H, et al. Effectiveness and safety of postoperative pain management: a survey of 18,925 consecutive patients between 1998 and 2006 (2nd revision): a database analysis of prospectively raised data. Br J Anaesth 2008;101(6):832–40.
8. Rodgers A, Walker N, Schug S, et al. Reduction of postoperative mortality and morbidity with epidural or spinal anaesthesia: results from overview of randomised trials. BMJ 2000;321(7275):1493.
9. Pöpping DM, Elia N, Van Aken HK, et al. Impact of epidural analgesia on mortality and morbidity after surgery: systematic review and meta-analysis of randomized controlled trials. Ann Surg 2014;259(6):1056–67.
10. Scott MJ, McEvoy MD, Gordon DB, et al. American Society for Enhanced Recovery (ASER) and perioperative quality initiative (POQI) joint consensus statement on optimal analgesia within an enhanced recovery pathway for colorectal surgery: part 2—from PACU to the transition home. Perioper Med (Lond) 2017;6(1):7.
11. Jorgensen H, Wetterslev J, Moiniche S, et al. Epidural local anaesthetics versus opioid-based analgesic regimens for postoperative gastrointestinal paralysis, PONV and pain after abdominal surgery. Cochrane Database Syst Rev 2001;(4):CD001893.
12. Fawcett WJ, Baldini G. Optimal analgesia during major open and laparoscopic abdominal surgery. Anesthesiol Clin 2015;33(1):65–78.
13. Liu H, Hu X, Duan X, et al. Thoracic epidural analgesia (TEA) vs. patient controlled analgesia (PCA) in laparoscopic colectomy: a meta-analysis. Hepatogastroenterology 2014;61(133):1213–9.
14. Hughes MJ, Ventham NT, McNally S, et al. Analgesia after open abdominal surgery in the setting of enhanced recovery surgery: a systematic review and meta-analysis. JAMA Surg 2014;149(12):1224–30.
15. Hübner M, Blanc C, Roulin D, et al. Randomized clinical trial on epidural versus patient-controlled analgesia for laparoscopic colorectal surgery within an enhanced recovery pathway. Ann Surg 2015;261(4):648–53.

16. Pirrera B, Alagna V, Lucchi A, et al. Transversus abdominis plane (TAP) block versus thoracic epidural analgesia (TEA) in laparoscopic colon surgery in the ERAS program. Surg Endosc 2018;32(1):376–82.
17. Szafran M. Role of regional analgesia. In: Gan TJ, Thacker JK, Miller TE, et al, editors. Enhanced recovery for major abdominopelvic surgery. American Society for Enhanced Recovery. Professional Communications, Inc; 2016. p. 165–76.
18. Meylan N, Elia N, Lysakowski C, et al. Benefit and risk of intrathecal morphine without local anaesthetic in patients undergoing major surgery: meta-analysis of randomized trials. Br J Anaesth 2009;102(2):156–67.
19. Koning MV, Teunissen AJW, Ruijgrok E, et al. Intrathecal morphine for laparoscopic segmental colonic resection as part of an enhanced recovery protocol: a randomized controlled trial. Reg Anesth pain Med 2018;43(2):166–73.
20. Levy B, Scott M, Fawcett W, et al. Randomized clinical trial of epidural, spinal or patient-controlled analgesia for patients undergoing laparoscopic colorectal surgery. Br J Surg 2011;98(8):1068–78.
21. Vaghadia H, Mcleod DH, Mitchell GE, et al. Small-dose hypobaric lidocaine-fentanyl spinal anesthesia for short duration outpatient laparoscopy. I. A randomized comparison with conventional dose hyperbaric lidocaine. Anesth Analg 1997;84(1):59–64.
22. Nimmo SM, Foo IT, Paterson HM. Enhanced recovery after surgery: pain management. J Surg Oncol 2017;116(5):583–91.
23. McDonnell JG, O'Donnell BD, Farrell T, et al. Transversus abdominis plane block: a cadaveric and radiological evaluation. Reg Anesth pain Med 2007;32(5):399–404.
24. Hebbard P. Subcostal transversus abdominis plane block under ultrasound guidance. Anesth Analg 2008;106(2):674–5.
25. McDonnell JG, O'donnell B, Curley G, et al. The analgesic efficacy of transversus abdominis plane block after abdominal surgery: a prospective randomized controlled trial. Anesth Analg 2007;104(1):193–7.
26. Hebbard P, Fujiwara Y, Shibata Y, et al. Ultrasound-guided transversus abdominis plane (TAP) block. Anaesth Intensive Care 2007;35(4):616–8.
27. Walter CJ, Maxwell-Armstrong C, Pinkney TD, et al. A randomised controlled trial of the efficacy of ultrasound-guided transversus abdominis plane (TAP) block in laparoscopic colorectal surgery. Surg Endosc 2013;27(7):2366–72.
28. Wu Y, Liu F, Tang H, et al. The analgesic efficacy of subcostal transversus abdominis plane block compared with thoracic epidural analgesia and intravenous opioid analgesia after radical gastrectomy. Anesth Analg 2013;117(2):507–13.
29. Park J-S, Choi G-S, Kwak K-H, et al. Effect of local wound infiltration and transversus abdominis plane block on morphine use after laparoscopic colectomy: a nonrandomized, single-blind prospective study. J Surg Res 2015;195(1):61–6.
30. Pedrazzani C, Menestrina N, Moro M, et al. Local wound infiltration plus transversus abdominis plane (TAP) block versus local wound infiltration in laparoscopic colorectal surgery and ERAS program. Surg Endosc 2016;30(11):5117–25.
31. Ortiz J, Suliburk JW, Wu K, et al. Bilateral transversus abdominis plane block does not decrease postoperative pain after laparoscopic cholecystectomy when compared with local anesthetic infiltration of trocar insertion sites. Reg Anesth pain Med 2012;37(2):188–92.
32. Kim AJ, Yong RJ, Urman RD. The role of transversus abdominis plane blocks in enhanced recovery after surgery pathways for open and laparoscopic colorectal surgery. J Laparoendosc Adv Surg Tech A 2017;27(9):909–14.
33. Ueshima H, Otake H, Lin J-A. Ultrasound-guided quadratus lumborum block: an updated review of anatomy and techniques. Biomed Res Int 2017;2017:2752876.

34. Elsayed H, McKevith J, McShane J, et al. Thoracic epidural or paravertebral catheter for analgesia after lung resection: is the outcome different? J Cardiothorac Vasc Anesth 2012;26(1):78–82.
35. Akcaboy EY, Akcaboy ZN, Gogus N. Comparison of paravertebral block versus fast-track general anesthesia via laryngeal mask airway in outpatient inguinal herniorrhaphy. J Anesth 2010;24(5):687–93.
36. Schnabel A, Reichl S, Kranke P, et al. Efficacy and safety of paravertebral blocks in breast surgery: a meta-analysis of randomized controlled trials. Br J Anaesth 2010;105(6):842–52.
37. El-Boghdadly K, Madjdpour C, Chin K. Thoracic paravertebral blocks in abdominal surgery: a systematic review of randomized controlled trials. Br J Anaesth 2016;117(3):297–308.
38. Møiniche S, Jørgensen H, Wetterslev J, et al. Local anesthetic infiltration for postoperative pain relief after laparoscopy: a qualitative and quantitative systematic review of intraperitoneal, port-site infiltration and mesosalpinx block. Anesth Analg 2000;90(4):899–912.
39. Afonso AM, Newman MI, Seeley N, et al. Multimodal analgesia in breast surgical procedures: technical and pharmacological considerations for liposomal bupivacaine use. Plast Reconstr Surg Glob Open 2017;5(9):e1480.
40. Stokes AL, Adhikary SD, Quintili A, et al. Liposomal bupivacaine use in transversus abdominis plane blocks reduces pain and postoperative intravenous opioid requirement after colorectal surgery. Dis Colon Rectum 2017;60(2):170–7.
41. McEvoy MD, Scott MJ, Gordon DB, et al. American Society for Enhanced Recovery (ASER) and perioperative quality initiative (POQI) joint consensus statement on optimal analgesia within an enhanced recovery pathway for colorectal surgery: part 1—from the preoperative period to PACU. Perioper Med (Lond) 2017;6(1):8.
42. Wu CL. Postoperative pain managment: enhanced recovery after major abdominopelvic surgery. In: Gan TJ, Thacker JK, Miller TE, et al, editors. Enhanced recovery for major abdominopelvic surgery. American Society for Enhanced Recovery. Professional Communications, Inc; 2016. p. 237–50.
43. De Oliveira GS Jr, Castro-Alves LJ, McCarthy RJ. Single-dose systemic acetaminophen to prevent postoperative pain: a meta-analysis of randomized controlled trials. Clin J pain 2015;31(1):86–93.
44. Doleman B, Read D, Lund JN, et al. Preventive acetaminophen reduces postoperative opioid consumption, vomiting, and pain scores after surgery: systematic review and meta-analysis. Reg Anesth pain Med 2015;40(6):706–12.
45. De Oliveira GS Jr, Agarwal D, Benzon HT. Perioperative single dose ketorolac to prevent postoperative pain: a meta-analysis of randomized trials. Anesth Analg 2012;114(2):424–33.
46. Marret E, Kurdi O, Zufferey P, et al. Effects of nonsteroidal antiinflammatory drugs on patient-controlled analgesia morphine side effects: meta-analysis of randomized controlled trials. Anesthesiology 2005;102(6):1249–60.
47. Straube S, Derry S, McQuay H, et al. Effect of preoperative Cox-II-selective NSAIDs (coxibs) on postoperative outcomes: a systematic review of randomized studies. Acta Anaesthesiol Scand 2005;49(5):601–13.
48. Maund E, McDaid C, Rice S, et al. Paracetamol and selective and non-selective non-steroidal anti-inflammatory drugs for the reduction in morphine-related side-effects after major surgery: a systematic review. Br J Anaesth 2011;106(3):292–7.
49. Michelet D, Andreu-Gallien J, Bensalah T, et al. A meta-analysis of the use of nonsteroidal antiinflammatory drugs for pediatric postoperative pain. Anesth Analg 2012;114(2):393–406.

50. Elia N, Lysakowski C, Tramèr MR. Does multimodal analgesia with acetaminophen, nonsteroidal antiinflammatory drugs, or selective cyclooxygenase-2 inhibitors and patient-controlled analgesia morphine offer advantages over morphine alone? Meta-analyses of randomized trials. Anesthesiology 2005;103(6):1296–304.
51. Cepeda MS, Carr DB, Miranda N, et al. Comparison of morphine, ketorolac, and their combination for postoperative pain results from a large, randomized, double-blind trial. Anesthesiology 2005;103(6):1225–32.
52. Gobble RM, Hoang HL, Kachniarz B, et al. Ketorolac does not increase periop-erative bleeding: a meta-analysis of randomized controlled trials. Plast Reconstr Surg 2014;133(3):741–55.
53. Leese PT, Hubbard RC, Karim A, et al. Effects of celecoxib, a novel cyclooxygenase-2 inhibitor, on platelet function in healthy adults: a randomized, controlled trial. J Clin Pharmacol 2000;40(2):124–32.
54. Subendran J, Siddiqui N, Victor JC, et al. NSAID use and anastomotic leaks following elective colorectal surgery: a matched case-control study. J Gastrointest Surg 2014;18(8):1391–7.
55. Saleh F, Jackson TD, Ambrosini L, et al. Perioperative nonselective non-steroidal anti-inflammatory drugs are not associated with anastomotic leakage after colo-rectal surgery. J Gastrointest Surg 2014;18(8):1398–404.
56. Van Koughnett JAM, Wexner SD. Surgery: NSAIDs and risk of anastomotic leaks after colorectal surgery. Nat Rev Gastroenterol Hepatol 2014;11(9):523.
57. Gorissen K, Benning D, Berghmans T, et al. Risk of anastomotic leakage with non-steroidal anti-inflammatory drugs in colorectal surgery. Br J Surg 2012;99(5):721–7.
58. Bhangu A, Singh P, Fitzgerald JEF, et al. Postoperative nonsteroidal anti-inflammatory drugs and risk of anastomotic leak: meta-analysis of clinical and experimental studies. World J Surg 2014;38(9):2247–57.
59. Hurley RW, Cohen SP, Williams KA, et al. The analgesic effects of perioperative gabapentin on postoperative pain: a meta-analysis. Reg Anesth pain Med 2006;31(3):237–47.
60. Mishriky B, Waldron N, Habib A. Impact of pregabalin on acute and persistent postoperative pain: a systematic review and meta-analysis. Br J Anaesth 2015;114(1):10–31.
61. Wang L, Johnston B, Kaushal A, et al. Ketamine added to morphine or hydromor-phone patient-controlled analgesia for acute postoperative pain in adults: a sys-tematic review and meta-analysis of randomized trials. Can J Anaesth 2016;63(3):311–25.
62. Loftus RW, Yeager MP, Clark JA, et al. Intraoperative ketamine reduces perioper-ative opiate consumption in opiate-dependent patients with chronic back pain undergoing back surgery. Anesthesiology 2010;113(3):639–46.
63. De Oliveira GS, Castro-Alves LJ, Khan JH, et al. Perioperative systemic magne-sium to minimize postoperative pain: a meta-analysis of randomized controlled trials. Anesthesiology 2013;119(1):178–90.
64. McCartney CJ, Sinha A, Katz J. A qualitative systematic review of the role of N-methyl-D-aspartate receptor antagonists in preventive analgesia. Anesth Analg 2004;98(5):1385–400.
65. Sun Y, Li T, Wang N, et al. Perioperative systemic lidocaine for postoperative anal-gesia and recovery after abdominal surgery: a meta-analysis of randomized controlled trials. Dis Colon Rectum 2012;55(11):1183–94.
66. Blaudszun G, Lysakowski C, Elia N, et al. Effect of perioperative systemic α2 ag-onists on postoperative morphine consumption and pain intensity: systematic

review and meta-analysis of randomized controlled trials. Anesthesiology 2012; 116(6):1312–22.

67. Jessen Lundorf L, Korvenius Nedergaard H, Møller A. Perioperative dexmedetomidine for acute pain after abdominal surgery in adults. Cochrane Database Syst Rev 2016;(2):CD010358.

68. Waldron N, Jones C, Gan T, et al. Impact of perioperative dexamethasone on postoperative analgesia and side-effects: systematic review and meta-analysis. Br J Anaesth 2013;110(2):191–200.

69. Tan E, Cornish J, Darzi A, et al. Meta-analysis: alvimopan vs. placebo in the treatment of post-operative ileus. Aliment Pharmacol Ther 2007;25(1):47–57.

70. Lee CT, Chang SS, Kamat AM, et al. Alvimopan accelerates gastrointestinal recovery after radical cystectomy: a multicenter randomized placebo-controlled trial. Eur Urol 2014;66(2):265–72.

Enhanced Recovery After Surgery
Intraoperative Fluid Management Strategies

Jeffrey W. Simmons, MD*, Jeffrey B. Dobyns, DO, MSHA, CMQ,
Juhan Paiste, MD, MBA

KEYWORDS

- ERAS • Fluid management • Goal-directed fluid therapy

KEY POINTS

- Intraoperative fluid management strategy should take into consideration surgery and patient risk.
- Goal-directed fluid therapy and restrictive fluid management are the most common strategies used in ERAS protocols.
- The goal of intraoperative fluid management is to maintain euvolemia.
- Both underresuscitation and overresuscitation have deleterious effects on patient outcome.
- Balanced salt solutions are better tolerated and should be the fluid of choice during crystalloid infusions.

INTRODUCTION

Enhanced recovery after surgery (ERAS) protocols incorporate a variety of perioperative interventions intending to preserve an individual's physiologic functions, alleviate surgical stress, and expedite recovery after surgery. One of the important, albeit frequently underappreciated and underused, components of any ERAS® protocol is optimal perioperative fluid management. Evidence suggests that changes in intraoperative fluid management alone can decrease postoperative complications by 50%.[1]

The essential objective of perioperative fluid management is to achieve a delicate balance between underresuscitation and overresuscitation. Underresuscitation results in hypovolemia-induced hypotension with impaired tissue perfusion and insufficient oxygenation. Overresuscitation results in volume overloaded cardiopulmonary complications, interstitial edema with gastrointestinal dysfunction, and anastomotic compromise.[2]

The authors have nothing to disclose.
Department of Anesthesiology and Perioperative Medicine, University of Alabama at Birmingham School of Medicine, JT 845, 619 South 19th Street, Birmingham, AL 35249, USA
* Corresponding author.
E-mail address: jwsimmons@uabmc.edu

Surg Clin N Am 98 (2018) 1185–1200
https://doi.org/10.1016/j.suc.2018.07.006   surgical.theclinics.com

For decades, liberal fluid management was the accepted canon for major surgical procedures. In their influential study from 1961, Shires and coworkers[3] concluded that loss of functional isotonic extracellular fluid in the first 2 hours of major surgery was independent of actual blood loss and was largely caused by internal redistribution. This became the theoretic foundation for "third-spacing" where extracellular fluid was contained in a transcellular space, neither intravascular, intracellular, nor interstitial. To manage third-spacing, liberal or conventional fluid management practices were used. Conventional management taught that surgical fluid replacement was a formula or recipe.

Total surgical crystalloid infusion =

1. Nothing by mouth (NPO; duration of NPO × maintenance fluid) +
2. Insensible losses (8 mL/kg/h for open abdominal procedure) +
3. Blood loss (3 × blood loss) +
4. Maintenance fluid (4 mL for 10-kg body weight, 2 mL for the second 10 kg, 1 mL for each subsequent 10 kg).

Using this formula, an 80-kg patient (NPO for 14 hours before surgery) having a 4-hour open abdominal procedure and 300 mL of blood loss would receive: maintenance fluid 120 mL/h (480 mL), NPO replacement (1680 mL), insensible losses (2560 mL), blood loss (900 mL), for a total of 5.6 L of crystalloid.

It was common practice for patients undergoing major abdominal surgery to be administered crystalloid infusions of 2 mL/kg/h to compensate for preoperative fasting and an additional volume of three to four times the actual blood loss.[4] Furthermore, insensible losses like third spacing, urine output, and evaporation were replaced at 4 to 8 mL/kg/h of crystalloid solution depending on incision size. These recommendations resulted in crystalloid infusion rates up to 20 mL/kg/h, if not higher. Infusion rates could be adjusted higher to maintain a urine output of 0.5 to 1 mL/kg/h.

Although liberal fluid management has been widely practiced, it has never been thoroughly studied.[5] Additionally, the myth of a third space has been largely debunked because of insufficient evidence of its existence through tracer studies.[6] It is now more commonly accepted to treat extracellular fluid as either intravascular or interstitial.

GOALS OF INTRAOPERATIVE FLUID MANAGEMENT IN ENHANCED RECOVERY AFTER SURGERY

The main objective of intraoperative fluid management is to preserve intravascular volume and at the same time avoid unnecessary salt and water intake through crystalloid solutions. Body fluid composition is divided into two compartments: intracellular and extracellular. Extracellular fluid is composed of plasma and interstitial fluid (**Fig. 1**). Interstitial dehydration and intravascular hypovolemia are distinctive clinical diagnoses that warrant different therapeutic considerations.[7] For example, insensible perspiration and urine production result in colloid-free fluid loss, but because of rapid redistribution between intravascular and interstitial spaces, the intravascular compartment is usually not directly affected. Thus, interstitial space replenishment by crystalloid solution administration can treat dehydration.[8,9] Contrary to dehydration, acute hypovolemia directly affects the intravascular compartment. Because crystalloid solutions diffuse freely between interstitial and intravascular space, they equilibrate rapidly and induce interstitial edema. Additionally, dilution of plasma with crystalloid solutions further decreases intravascular oncotic pressure and facilitates fluid shifting into interstitial space. Thus, a euvolemic state is achieved through a delicate balance of maintenance fluid and volume-replacement therapy.

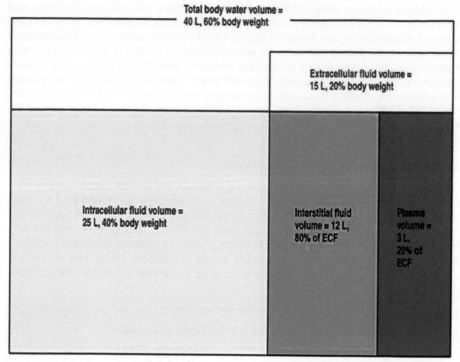

Fig. 1. Body fluid composition. ECF, extracellular fluid.

Maintenance fluid administration is intended to replace losses associated with insensible perspiration and urine production, which are frequently less than ordinarily thought. This fluid requirement is achieved by balanced crystalloid solution delivered at 1 to 3 mL/kg/h.[9] This approach has also been called restrictive or "zero-balance fluid therapy."

Volume-replacement therapy is required to treat hypovolemia caused by surgical blood loss and/or intravascular volume shift into interstitial place. In case intravascular hypovolemia is suspected, the recommended approach is to administer a fluid challenge to test cardiovascular system responsiveness to increased intravascular volume (by shifting the Frank-Starling curve to the right). It is recommended that this fluid challenge be given promptly over 5 to 10 minutes.[10] A point of consideration is that intraoperative hemodynamic instability cannot always be attributed to hypovolemia because only about 50% of intraoperative hemodynamically unstable patients are "fluid-challenge" responsive.[11]

INFUSION STRATEGIES

Fluid therapy in any perioperative protocol should be patient-centric, evidence-based, with consideration of physiologic principles and local expertise. Anesthesiologists should formulate a patient-specific plan for fluid optimization and monitoring based on specific comorbidities and degree of surgical risk.[12]

Conventional or Liberal Fluid Management

In the setting of ambulatory surgery with low-risk patients undergoing low-risk procedures, liberal fluid strategies using crystalloid infusions up to 20 to 30 mL/kg/h may reduce postoperative dizziness, drowsiness, pain, nausea and vomiting, and length of stay in the ambulatory center.[12] A study from 2004 examining American Society of Anesthesiologists Physical Status I or II patients undergoing laparoscopic cholecystectomy found that patients who received 40 mL/kg of intraoperative fluid experienced improvement in pulmonary function, exercise capacity, and general well-being, along with decreased hospitalization.[13] Although these low-risk patient and procedure studies, such as laparoscopic cholecystectomy or herniorrhaphy, have demonstrated benefits from liberal fluid management, the results cannot be extrapolated to patients, either low- or high-risk, undergoing major and more extensive intra-abdominal procedures.[14]

Zero-Balance or Restrictive Fluid Management

As patients and procedures transition from lower- to higher-risk classifications, fluid management becomes increasingly complex. In these patients, liberal fluid administration is associated with worsened outcomes. Restrictive fluid management replaces blood loss on a milliliter-for-milliliter basis with colloid and minimal to no maintenance crystalloid rate for insensible losses. Appropriateness of patients to receive restrictive fluid management should be determined based on patient health status and risk coupled with procedural risk, as demonstrated by **Table 1**. Higher-risk patients,

Table 1
Determination of appropriate patients for restrictive fluid management

	Low Patient Risk MACE Risk <1%[a]	High Patient Risk MACE Risk >1%[a]
Low procedural risk[b]	Monitors • Standard ASA Fluid strategy • Liberal[12] • Zero-balance Fluid choice • Balanced salt crystalloid	Monitors • Standard ASA • Noninvasive cardiac output monitor • Esophageal Doppler • ± Arterial line Fluid strategy • Goal-directed Fluid choice • Colloid with balanced salt crystalloid
Elevated procedural risk[b]	Monitors • Standard ASA • ± Arterial line Fluid strategy • Restrictive Fluid choice • Balanced salt crystalloid	Monitors • Standard ASA • Arterial line • Noninvasive cardiac output monitor • TEE/TTE Fluid strategy • Goal-directed Fluid choice • Colloid with balanced salt crystalloid

Elevated risk: anticipated increased blood loss greater than 500 mL; aortic, carotid, or peripheral vascular surgery; abdominal or thoracic surgery; head and neck surgery; major orthopedic surgery; prostate surgery.
    Low risk: anticipated low blood loss less than 500 mL, breast surgery, cataract surgery, superficial surgery, endoscopy, minor orthopedic surgery.
    Abbreviations: ASA, American Society of Anesthesiologists; MACE, major adverse cardiovascular event; TEE, transesophageal echocardiography; TTE, transthoracic echocardiography.
    [a] MACE risk: based on Gupta Perioperative Cardiac Risk Calculator.
    [b] Procedural risk categories.[81]
    Data from Navarro LH, Bloomstone JA, Auler JO Jr, et al. Perioperative fluid therapy: a statement from the international Fluid Optimization Group. Perioper Med (Lond) 2015;4:3.

such as those with heart failure, may acutely decompensate from fluid boluses and would likely benefit from having fluids titrated to specific hemodynamic targets.

Goal-Directed Fluid Therapy

Excessive fluid administration in high-risk patients results in life-threatening complications, such as pulmonary edema and death. Goal-directed fluid management, in which intravenous fluid is administered to attain a specific target, such as stroke volume or cardiac index, results in reduced perioperative morbidity and duration of hospitalization. Goal-directed fluid therapy (GDFT) involves the administration of small-volume (100–250 mL) colloid boluses rather than maintenance crystalloid infusion (3–4 mL/kg/h) titrated to maintain stroke volume and cardiac output.[14,15] Although outcomes are improved, the results of the OPTIMISE Trial found no direct reduction of 30-day mortality in high-risk patients compared with "usual" non-goal-directed therapy. When this trial was included in an updated meta-analysis, GDFT was associated with reduced overall complications.[16,17] It should be noted that ERAS protocols traditionally rely on restrictive management strategies or GDFT.

Preoperative Testing

Health care expenditures directed toward preoperative testing are significant, and reduction in unnecessary testing is estimated nationally to save $10 billion annually.[18] Eliminating unnecessary preoperative testing decreases health care costs, improves quality, and enhances patient satisfaction. Preoperative testing should be patient-centered and determined by patient health status and functional capacity. Although no laboratory studies can identify which patients may or may not be appropriate for restrictive fluid therapy, the development of individualized fluid-management plans should consider patient risk for perioperative adverse outcomes according to a verified major adverse cardiovascular event scoring system. Commonly used major adverse cardiovascular event scoring systems are Gupta Perioperative Cardiac Risk or Lee Revised Cardiac Risk Index. Patient's with elevated major adverse cardiovascular event scores ($\geq$1%) should be considered at elevated risk and be stratified to receive GDFT or restrictive fluid management. Alternatively, the measurement of certain biomarkers, such as brain natriuretic peptide or N-terminal fragment of pro–brain natriuretic peptide, may be used to risk stratify patients.[19] Preoperative troponin measurements have also been used to predict postsurgical complications.[20] When appropriate, the combined approach to risk stratification allows for precise stratification and inclusion into the correct fluid management strategy.

PERIOPERATIVE FLUID SELECTION

The therapeutic effect of intravenous fluid administration results from expansion of the intravascular, interstitial, or intracellular compartments. Fluid resuscitation is indicated for intravascular and extravascular hypovolemia that causes hemodynamic instability manifesting as end-organ hypoperfusion, dehydration, and hyperosmolarity.[21]

Perioperative fluid selection directly affects postoperative outcomes. The choice of colloid versus crystalloid for resuscitation is a continuing debate. Compared with crystalloid resuscitation, colloid use provides a more efficient plasma volume expansion with lower volumes.[22] Optimal fluid management in ERAS uses a balanced approach with crystalloids and colloids titrated to hemodynamic stability and urine output maintenance of 0.5 mL/kg/h.[23] Maintenance crystalloid fluids, when used, should be restricted to less than 2 mL/kg/h, accounting for volume associated with drug infusions.

Crystalloids

Normal saline

Large volumes of normal saline (NS) infusion result in hypernatremia and hyperchloremic metabolic acidemia. Hyperchloremia produces renal vasoconstriction and decreased cortical perfusion, leading to acute kidney injury (AKI), increased length of hospitalization, and 30-day mortality.[21,24–26] NS is not recommended as a perioperative fluid for these reasons. The use of NS versus balanced salt solutions in neurosurgery is debatable and beyond the scope of discussion.

Balanced salt solutions

Balanced salt solutions, such as lactated Ringers, NormoSol, and Plasmalyte, have shown no adverse effects in any patient population.[21] They are not associated with hyperchloremia or hypernatremia and are the recommended perioperative fluid. Gastrointestinal dysfunction and delayed bowel recovery are two commonly described postoperative complications of large-volume crystalloid infusions.[22]

Colloids

Gelatins

Gelatins are protein-based colloids derived from bovine collagen. Concerns about Creutzfeldt-Jacob disease and bovine spongiform encephalitis have limited their use. None of the three commercially available gelatins are available in the United States, having been removed from use in 1978 because of a high incidence of hypersensitivity reactions.[27] Although gelatins purportedly have few adverse side effects, recent studies have shown a negative effect on thromboelastography and should be used cautiously in patients with disorders of hemostasis.[28] Additionally, gelatin usage was associated with a heightened risk of AKI.[29]

Dextrans

Dextran is a polysaccharide molecule available in different molecular weights. Dextrans have excellent volume expansion properties, but reduce platelet aggregation and adhesiveness leading to a von Willebrand–like syndrome and increased fibrinolysis, the severity of which is increased with higher molecular weight dextrans. They also have a high incidence of immunogenic and nonimmunogenic hypersensitivity reactions. An increase in acute renal failure in patients with stroke treated with dextrans has also been described.[27] They are expensive and current recommendations are to limit doses to 1500 mL/d in adult and 20 mL/kg in pediatric patients. Current literature suggests benefit from pretreatment against anaphylaxis before use.[27]

Hydroxyethyl starch

Hydroxyethyl starches (HES) are plant-based starches with a large carbohydrate molecule as the colloid base. Older-generation HES products are known for accumulation in skin, kidney, or liver, resulting in organ dysfunction, such as AKI, acute portal hypertension and liver failure, and protracted pruritis.[30–33] HES are also associated with decreased function of von Willebrand factor, factor VIII, and platelets, although this effect is less with newer generation solutions.[27] These adverse coagulation effects were substantiated in a meta-analysis from 2001 that demonstrated increased blood loss compared with albumin in patients undergoing cardiopulmonary bypass.[34] Despite these concerns, HES continue to be widely used. Current recommendations are to limit dosage to 33 to 50 mL/kg/d.[29]

Blood Products

Anemia is a common perioperative problem, affecting 30% to 50% of patients presenting for cardiac and noncardiac surgery, and is associated with increased 30-day morbidity and mortality.[35–37] It is also potentially treatable. A large observational study found that preoperative and early postoperative anemia were directly correlated with AKI.[38]

Medical management

Correction of perioperative anemia should occur based on its cause. Iron, folate, vitamin B_{12} supplementation, or erythrocyte-stimulating medications can be used as appropriate. Management of perioperative anemia should occur over 3 to 4 weeks.

Blood transfusion

Blood transfusion rapidly corrects anemia and is appropriate for patients with severe and symptomatic anemia or those undergoing large-volume blood loss procedures. Blood transfusion should be used cautiously and sparingly, because of an association with a dose-dependent increase in morbidity and mortality.[39,40] Packed red blood cells and fresh frozen plasma are not indicated for routine volume expansion in the absence of symptomatic anemia or tissue hypoxia related to decreased oxygen-carrying capacity. In addition, transfusion of fresh frozen plasma carries infection risk. Although transfusion can indeed be life-saving, significant volume expansion and peripheral edema results with expected complications, such as immunosuppression, transfusion-related reactions, and poor wound healing.[41] Liberal (maintenance of hemoglobin 10–12 g/dL) versus restrictive (maintenance of hemoglobin 7–9 g/dL) transfusion triggers are beyond the scope of discussion, except to note that liberal transfusion approaches were associated with increased poor clinical outcomes.[42]

END POINTS OF RESUSCITATION FOR GOAL-DIRECTED FLUID THERAPY

Classical end points of resuscitation, such as urine output, heart rate, and blood pressure, suffice for most healthy ERAS patients. Protocolized fluid strategies with fixed infusion volumes per hour are simple and promote high compliance (500 mL/h for laparoscopy; 800 mL/h for open laparotomy). When a patient is having more complex surgery with increased risk for bleeding or has a complex medical history, the use of GDFT becomes paramount to decrease surgical morbidity and intensive care unit days (see **Table 1**).[43] Interestingly, the use of GDFT has a stronger relationship with reduction in morbidity when used outside of ERAS protocols versus when used with ERAS protocols.[44] GDFT uses dynamic markers to predict fluid responsiveness, such as pulse pressure and stroke volume variation (PPV), cardiac output index, and systemic vascular resistance index. GDFT is thus a modality to ensure proper placement on the Frank-Starling curve. Commonly used GDFT modalities in ERAS include noninvasive cardiac output, transesophageal Doppler (TED), and arterial line monitoring. Comparing liberal fluid therapy with GDFT, high-risk patients receiving GDFT have less risk of pneumonia, less pulmonary edema, reduced length of hospital stay, and earlier return of bowel function. Mortality, wound infections, and renal failure were not significantly different between the two groups.[45]

Noninvasive Cardiac Output Monitoring

Bioreactance is a method for noninvasive cardiac output monitoring that uses external electrode pads placed on the skin of the abdomen and chest. Using low-amplitude, high-frequency electrical current, phase shifts are measured that correlate to the degree of volume resuscitation. The premise of bioreactance measuring devices is that with greater stroke volumes, greater phase shifts occur.[46] Bioreactance devices (Cheetah Medical, Newton Center, MA) are capable of measuring cardiac output index, stroke volume index, and variation, and derive peripheral vascular resistance.

The electrodes may be used continuously from surgery to the postoperative period for high-risk patients (see **Table 1**). Weaknesses of these devices are that the electrode pads must be positioned outside of the surgical site and have significant disruption by electrocautery. A recent prospective comparison between TED monitoring and Cheetah noninvasive cardiac output monitoring revealed consistent correlation between the two devices with no differences in clinical outcomes of length of stay.[47]

Transesophageal Doppler

TED measurements of cardiac output are derived from blood flow in the descending aorta. A small probe is placed in the esophagus that continuously measures red blood cell velocity in the adjacent descending aorta.[48] Predicting fluid responsiveness is possible by bolusing 200 to 500 mL of crystalloid and assessing the changed in stoke volume. An increase of more than 10% indicates possible responsiveness to additional fluid.[44] The esophageal Doppler has benefits of easy placements in the anesthetized patient; however, it may move within the esophagus requiring careful attention to location. Guinot and coworkers[49] evaluated the ability of TED to predict fluid responsiveness in 90 patients and found that at change in stroke volume variation of greater than 14% after 500 mL fluid challenge most accurately predicted responsiveness to additional fluid. A meta-analysis of nine clinical trials (seven in surgery, two in intensive care unit) using TED revealed significant reduction in post-procedure length of stay (2.17–2.34 reduction).[50] Placement of the probe using the nasopharyngeal approach is better tolerated in the awake patient and is used for postoperative monitoring in high-risk patients (see **Table 1**).

Pulse Pressure/Stroke Volume Variation

Using an arterial catheter for monitoring hemodynamics is reasonable in high-risk patients or patients undergoing high-risk for bleeding surgery (see **Table 1**). With specialized software or external modules, such as the Vigileo Monitor (Edwards Lifesciences, Irvine, CA), PPV is obtained. Multiple studies have confirmed the validity of pulse pressure variation to predict fluid responsiveness.[51–54] Confounding the of use PPV is that it directly correlates with the tidal volume delivered by mechanical ventilation.[54] Larger tidal volumes increase the change in pulse pressure. Using lung protective ventilation strategies of 6 to 8 mL/kg of ideal body weight for tidal volumes minimizes the variance in pulse pressure. Open chest procedures also decrease the variation when using PPV making it less useful in thoracic surgery. The benefits of PPV monitoring in major abdominal or gynecologic surgery are as described for any GDFT management, but with the ability to sample arterial blood for markers of adequate microcirculation, such as lactate and base deficit.

PATHOPHYSIOLOGY OF INAPPROPRIATE FLUID RESUSCITATION IN SURGERY

Oliguria following anesthesia and surgery is common and the associated differential diagnosis is lengthy. Although oliguria should trigger diagnostic efforts, fluid therapy is not indicated until hypovolemia is confirmed as the cause.[55] Although hypovolemia and hypervolemia are detrimental, numerous studies demonstrate that excess fluid administration causes postoperative complications, such as increased hospitalization and risk of death after surgery.[56–60] Furthermore, there is an observed correlation between perioperative increase in body weight and postoperative complications (**Fig. 2**).

Overresuscitation

Positive fluid balance, defined as 10% or greater increase in weight perioperatively, is associated with increased complications and mortality in medical and surgical

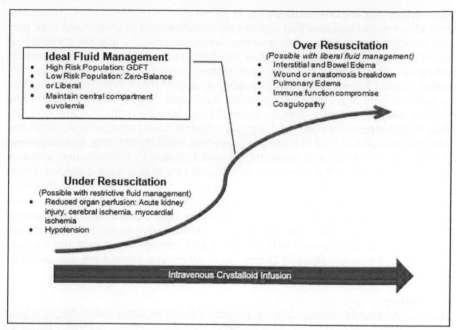

Fig. 2. Resuscitation curve.

patients.[61] Intravascular fluid overload causing weight gain is specifically associated with greater morbidity following colorectal surgery. Excess fluid volume contributes to cardiac dysfunction, pulmonary edema, bowel edema, adynamic ileus, and associated postoperative nausea and vomiting. Furthermore, excessive intravenous fluid administration impairs tissue oxygenation, induces hypoxia, and undermines the healing process.[59]

Bowel edema

Excessive fluid administration leads to bowel edema, which contributes to enteric nutritional intolerance, prolonged ileus, and endotoxin or gut bacteria translocation, with the potentially significant sequelae of sepsis and multiorgan failure.[62] Bowel edema is more likely following administration of crystalloids as opposed to colloids and may result in increased tension at anastomotic sites leading to anastomotic dehiscence, peritoneal contamination, sepsis, and death.[62]

Wound healing

Subcutaneous edema leads to decreased tissue oxygen diffusion and oxygen tension resulting in poor wound healing. Goal-directed crystalloid administration resulted in a greater concentration of collagen in surgical wounds.[63] GDFT using 6% HES compared with crystalloid-based fluid therapy resulted in improved microcirculatory blood flow and tissue oxygenation at colonic anastomotic sites in animal studies.[64]

Pulmonary complications

Excessive fluid administration leads to pulmonary edema, particularly in heart failure patients. Increased extravascular lung water impairs oxygen exchange leading to respiratory failure and pneumonia.[62] Pulmonary edema has been described because of fluid overload even for patients without preexisting cardiac disease.[65,66]

Inflammatory and immune response

It has also been suggested that liberal perioperative fluid management may promote infections; excessive cell swelling weakens immune system because of impaired lymphocyte signaling.[67] It is not disputed that postoperative immune dysfunction predisposes patients to a higher incidence of complications.[68–70] Several studies have further demonstrated a relationship between the selection and administered amount of perioperative fluids and degree of inflammation and effect on cellular immunity. A study from 2014 comparing restrictive and conventional fluid therapies in colorectal surgery patients found that patients receiving restrictive amounts of fluid had greater preserved cellular immunity, as determined by $CD4^+/CD8^+$ ratios and regulatory T-cell function.[71] Furthermore, patients receiving conventional fluid therapy had a higher rate of blood transfusions. Blood transfusions are themselves immunosuppressant, the effects being cumulative. Regarding fluid choice, hyperchloremic metabolic acidosis is associated with a proinflammatory response and decreased immunologic function.[72] In an animal study looking at a rat model of sepsis, survival rates were better for resuscitative fluids consisting of balanced salt solutions and colloids (here lactated Ringers and HES) than with NS alone.[73] This collectively argues against the use of NS as a perioperative resuscitative fluid.

Coagulopathy

Excessive crystalloid infusion during surgery influences coagulation negatively at different stages. Dilutional thrombocytopenia remains the most common cause of intraoperative bleeding. Colloids, particularly the starches, have been associated with decreased coagulation, such as HES-mediated reduction of factor VIII and von Willebrand factor, and are discussed in greater detail later.[74] Crystalloid and colloid solutions administered intraoperatively in the trauma setting may induce coagulopathy because of dilution, acidosis, or accelerated thrombolysis.[75] This is more prominent when hypotension or shock is present.[76] Postoperatively, evidence suggests that crystalloid dilution of anticoagulatory factors results in a hypercoagulable state leading to thromboembolic consequences.[62,74,77]

Underresuscitation

Hypovolemia may result in poor tissue perfusion, end-organ dysfunction and failure, and ultimately death.

Acute kidney injury

Although 1% to 5% of hospital admissions experience AKI, it is particularly ominous perioperatively where it portends a more complex hospital course with increased health care costs and high morbidity and mortality. AKI necessitating dialysis is an independent risk factor for death.[78] The most significant perioperative factor for prevention of AKI is the maintenance of normal renal perfusion using GDFT to achieve and maintain normovolemia.

Hypotension

Underresuscitation leads to hypovolemia, hypotension, and impaired end-organ perfusion. Mean arterial pressures less than 55 mm Hg directly correlate with postoperative AKI.[79] Monitoring of urine output is frequently undertaken as a means of monitoring volume status and hypotension with an accompanying decrease in urine output may prompt administration of fluid boluses. Because of complex neuroendocrine factors and pathways, urine output is poorly responsive to fluid boluses, and this therapy risks excessive fluid administration.

STANDARDIZING FLUID MANAGEMENT: HOW CAN IT BE DONE CONSISTENTLY?

To achieve high compliance with ERAS intraoperative fluid management, the first step is to collaboratively agree on management protocols and defined end points specific to the service line or procedure. End points of resuscitation necessarily differ between different service lines and procedures. The process begins by choosing surgical and anesthesia "champions" and assembling key perioperative personnel (preoperative and postoperative nursing, nurse anesthesia, preoperative assessment clinic representation). Evidence-based protocols are constructed with input from the team, creating early buy-in and acceptance. Perioperative representation is essential because fluid management begins before the patient arrives to surgery (bowel preparation, NPO status, preoperative hydration) and continues into the postoperative period. Management goals for a procedure should be clearly defined, avoiding such general terms as restrictive or liberal. For example, open colectomy 800 mL/h, laparoscopic colectomy 400 mL/h is more practical to the end-user and simpler to audit. The protocol is then made available to faculty and staff in useable formats (paper, World Wide Web–based, telephone application, or embedded into the electronic medical record). Next, identification of the patient as an ERAS patient is crucial to success. This is done by attaching ERAS to the anesthesia type requested (ERAS + general) or attaching ERAS to the surgical procedure name (ERAS colectomy). Inserting the patient's ERAS status into the surgical time out is also a known focal point for most surgeries. Next, regular audits are necessary to measure compliance and identify weak points. Audits, whether electronic or manual, should occur regularly and be transparent for the perioperative team. These audits can also be placed into an ERAS scorecard allowing the surgeon or anesthesiologist to visualize their performance. Finally, the perioperative team should reconvene after implementation to study outcomes and determine if revision is necessary. Fluid management strategies from different institutions are accessed at the American Society of Enhanced Recovery (http://aserhq.org) or ERAS® Society (http://erassociety.org) Web sites.

SUMMARY

ERAS protocols use best practice, evidence-based elements, such as GDFT, to mitigate the stress of surgery, reduce surgical complications, and shorten hospital length of stay. Perioperative fluid management strategies are a customary component of successful surgery with the preoperative management affecting the intraoperative management and so on. Equally as important, the elements of an ERAS protocol are collaboratively established between anesthesia and surgery to facilitate a team approach where members can rely on consistent care. For low-risk patients having low-risk surgery, liberal fluid management has not been shown to compromise successful outcomes. Conversely, GDFT in high-risk surgical patients or those having major surgery has greater benefit and is associated with improved surgical outcomes. Reductions in hospital length of stay, improved return of bowel function, and protection of bowel anastomosis are evident in major surgical procedures when using GDFT. Although the use of GDFT has unquestioned benefit in certain surgeries, several questions still remain regarding the ideal end point for fluid resuscitation, type of resuscitation fluid, the best monitoring technology, and the ideal population for GDFT.[80] Trials evaluating GDFT have not been consistent, using different end points, different interventions, and different monitors.[60] These unanswered questions often lead to great variability that leads to nonstandardized care. Variability in care is the antithesis of an ERAS protocol. By incorporating concrete fluid management guidelines into a local ERAS protocol, consistency and compliance are more readily achieved.

Monitoring practice patterns within the electronic medical records and issuing providers with monthly reports accelerate compliance especially when patient-centered outcomes are tied to practice patterns.

REFERENCES

1. Brandstrup B, Tonnesen H, Beier-Holgersen R, et al. Effects of intravenous fluid restriction on postoperative complications: comparison of two perioperative fluid regimens: a randomized assessor-blinded multicenter trial. Ann Surg 2003; 238(5):641–8.
2. Brandstrup B. Fluid therapy for the surgical patient. Best Pract Res Clin Anaesthesiol 2006;20(2):265–83.
3. Shires T, Williams J, Brown F. Acute change in extracellular fluids associated with major surgical procedures. Ann Surg 1961;154:803–10.
4. Bamboat ZM, Bordeianou L. Perioperative fluid management. Clin Colon Rectal Surg 2009;22(1):28–33.
5. Hannemann P, Lassen K, Hausel J, et al. Patterns in current anaesthesiological peri-operative practice for colonic resections: a survey in five northern-European countries. Acta Anaesthesiol Scand 2006;50(9):1152–60.
6. Jacob M, Chappell D, Rehm M. The 'third space': fact or fiction? Best Pract Res Clin Anaesthesiol 2009;23(2):145–57.
7. Miller TE, Roche AM, Mythen M. Fluid management and goal-directed therapy as an adjunct to enhanced recovery after surgery (ERAS). Can J Anaesth 2015; 62(2):158–68.
8. Strunden MS, Heckel K, Goetz AE, et al. Perioperative fluid and volume management: physiological basis, tools and strategies. Ann Intensive Care 2011;1(1):2.
9. Chappell D, Jacob M, Hofmann-Kiefer K, et al. A rational approach to perioperative fluid management. Anesthesiology 2008;109(4):723–40.
10. Cecconi M, Parsons AK, Rhodes A. What is a fluid challenge? Curr Opin Crit Care 2011;17(3):290–5.
11. Marik PE, Lemson J. Fluid responsiveness: an evolution of our understanding. Br J Anaesth 2014;112(4):617–20.
12. Navarro LH, Bloomstone JA, Auler JO Jr, et al. Perioperative fluid therapy: a statement from the international Fluid Optimization Group. Perioper Med (Lond) 2015;4:3.
13. Holte K, Klarskov B, Christensen DS, et al. Liberal versus restrictive fluid administration to improve recovery after laparoscopic cholecystectomy: a randomized, double-blind study. Ann Surg 2004;240(5):892–9.
14. Nisanevich V, Felsenstein I, Almogy G, et al. Effect of intraoperative fluid management on outcome after intraabdominal surgery. Anesthesiology 2005;103(1):25–32.
15. Biais M, de Courson H, Lanchon R, et al. Mini-fluid challenge of 100 ml of crystalloid predicts fluid responsiveness in the operating room. Anesthesiology 2017; 127(3):450–6.
16. Pearse R, Dawson D, Fawcett J, et al. Early goal-directed therapy after major surgery reduces complications and duration of hospital stay. A randomized controlled trial. Crit Care 2005;9:R687–93.
17. Pearse RM, Harrison DA, MacDonald N, et al. Effect of a perioperative, cardiac output-guided hemodynamic therapy algorithm on outcomes following major gastrointestinal surgery: a randomized clinical trial and systematic review. JAMA 2014;311(21):2181–90.
18. Brown SR, Brown J. Why do physicians order unnecessary preoperative tests? A qualitative study. Fam Med 2011;43(5):338–43.

19. Duceppe E, Parlow J, MacDonald P, et al. Canadian Cardiovascular Society guidelines on perioperative cardiac risk assessment and management for patients who undergo noncardiac surgery. Can J Cardiol 2017;33(1):17–32.
20. Maile MD, Jewell ES, Engoren MC. Timing of preoperative troponin elevations and postoperative mortality after noncardiac surgery. Anesth Analg 2016;123(1):135–40.
21. Lira A, Pinsky M. Choices in fluid type and volume during resuscitation: impact on patient outcomes. Ann Intensive Care 2014;4(38):1–13.
22. Gan TJ. Colloid or crystalloid: any differences in outcomes? Presented at the IARS annual meeting held at Vancouver, British Columbia, Canada on May 21–24, 2011. p. 7–12. Available at: http://iars.org/wp-content/uploads/2011_IARS_Review_Course_Lectures.pdf. Accessed August 13, 2018.
23. Joshi GP. Intraoperative fluid restriction improves outcome after major elective gastrointestinal surgery. Anesth Analg 2005;101(2):601–5.
24. McCluskey SA, Karkouti K, Wijeysundera D, et al. Hyperchloremia after noncardiac surgery is independently associated with increased morbidity and mortality: a propensity-matched cohort study. Anesth Analg 2013;117(2):412–21.
25. Feldheiser A, Aziz O, Baldini G, et al. Enhanced recovery after surgery (ERAS) for gastrointestinal surgery, part 2: consensus statement for anaesthesia practice. Acta Anaesthesiol Scand 2016;60(3):289–334.
26. Chowdhury AH, Cox EF, Francis ST, et al. A randomized, controlled, double-blind crossover study on the effects of 2-L infusions of 0.9% saline and plasma-lyte(R) 148 on renal blood flow velocity and renal cortical tissue perfusion in healthy volunteers. Ann Surg 2012;256(1):18–24.
27. Bailey A, McNaull P, Jooste E, et al. Perioperative crystalloid and colloid fluid management in children: where are we and how did we get here? Anesth Analg 2010;110(2):375–90.
28. de Jonge E, Levi M. Effects of different plasma substitutes on blood coagulation: a comparative review. Crit Care Med 2001;29(6):1261–7.
29. Myburgh JA, Mythen MG. Resuscitation fluids. N Engl J Med 2013;369(13):1243–51.
30. Wiedermann CJ, Joannidis M. Accumulation of hydroxyethyl starch in human and animal tissues: a systematic review. Intensive Care Med 2014;40(2):160–70.
31. Christidis C, Mal F, Ramos J, et al. Worsening of hepatic dysfunction as a consequence of repeated hydroxyethylstarch infusions. J Hepatol 2001;35(6):726–32.
32. Bork K. Pruritus precipitated by hydroxyethyl starch: a review. Br J Dermatol 2005;152(1):3–12.
33. Zarychanski R, Abou-Setta AM, Turgeon AF, et al. Association of hydroxyethyl starch administration with mortality and acute kidney injury in critically ill patients requiring volume resuscitation: a systematic review and meta-analysis. JAMA 2013;309(7):678–88.
34. Wilkes MM, Navickis RJ, Sibbald WJ. Albumin versus hydroxyethyl starch in cardiopulmonary bypass surgery: a meta-analysis of postoperative bleeding. Ann Thorac Surg 2001;72(2):527–33 [discussion: 534].
35. Horres CR, Adam MA, Sun Z, et al. Proceedings of the American Society for Enhanced Recovery/evidence based perioperative medicine 2016 annual congress of enhanced recovery and perioperative medicine. Perioper Med (Lond) 2016;5(Suppl 1):1–13.
36. Musallam KM, Tamim HM, Richards T, et al. Preoperative anaemia and postoperative outcomes in non-cardiac surgery: a retrospective cohort study. Lancet 2011;378(9800):1396–407.

37. Hung M, Besser M, Sharples LD, et al. The prevalence and association with transfusion, intensive care unit stay and mortality of pre-operative anaemia in a cohort of cardiac surgery patients. Anaesthesia 2011;66(9):812–8.
38. Walsh M, Garg A, Devereaux P, et al. The association between perioperative hemoglobin and acute kidney injury in patients having noncardiac surgery. Anesth Analg 2013;117:924–31.
39. Bernard AC, Davenport DL, Chang PK, et al. Intraoperative transfusion of 1 U to 2 U packed red blood cells is associated with increased 30-day mortality, surgical-site infection, pneumonia, and sepsis in general surgery patients. J Am Coll Surg 2009;208(5):931–7, 937.e1–2; [discussion: 938-9].
40. Refaai MA, Blumberg N. The transfusion dilemma: weighing the known and newly proposed risks of blood transfusions against the uncertain benefits. Best Pract Res Clin Anaesthesiol 2013;27(1):17–35.
41. Hare GM, Baker JE, Pavenski K. Assessment and treatment of preoperative anemia: continuing professional development. Can J Anaesth 2011;58(6):569–81.
42. Moemen M. Fluid therapy: too much or too little. Egypt J Anaesth 2010;26:313–8.
43. Benes J, Giglio M, Brienza N, et al. The effects of goal-directed fluid therapy based on dynamic parameters on post-surgical outcome: a meta-analysis of randomized controlled trials. Crit Care 2014;18(5):584.
44. Rollins KE, Lobo DN. Intraoperative goal-directed fluid therapy in elective major abdominal surgery: a meta-analysis of randomized controlled trials. Ann Surg 2016;263(3):465–76.
45. Corcoran T, Rhodes JE, Clarke S, et al. Perioperative fluid management strategies in major surgery: a stratified meta-analysis. Anesth Analg 2012;114(3):640–51.
46. Fagnoul D, Vincent JL, Backer de D. Cardiac output measurements using the bioreactance technique in critically ill patients. Crit Care 2012;16(6):460.
47. Waldron NH, Miller TE, Thacker JK, et al. A prospective comparison of a noninvasive cardiac output monitor versus esophageal Doppler monitor for goal-directed fluid therapy in colorectal surgery patients. Anesth Analg 2014;118(5): 966–75.
48. Cecconi M, De Backer D, Antonelli M, et al. Consensus on circulatory shock and hemodynamic monitoring. task force of the European Society of Intensive Care Medicine. Intensive Care Med 2014;40(12):1795–815.
49. Guinot PG, de Broca B, Abou Arab O, et al. Ability of stroke volume variation measured by oesophageal Doppler monitoring to predict fluid responsiveness during surgery. Br J Anaesth 2013;110(1):28–33.
50. Phan TD, Ismail H, Heriot AG, et al. Improving perioperative outcomes: fluid optimization with the esophageal Doppler monitor, a metaanalysis and review. J Am Coll Surg 2008;207(6):935–41.
51. Theerawit P, Morasert T, Sutherasan Y. Inferior vena cava diameter variation compared with pulse pressure variation as predictors of fluid responsiveness in patients with sepsis. J Crit Care 2016;36:246–51.
52. Lopes MR, Oliveira MA, Pereira VO, et al. Goal-directed fluid management based on pulse pressure variation monitoring during high-risk surgery: a pilot randomized controlled trial. Crit Care 2007;11(5):R100.
53. Piccioni F, Bernasconi F, Tramontano GT, et al. A systematic review of pulse pressure variation and stroke volume variation to predict fluid responsiveness during cardiac and thoracic surgery. J Clin Monit Comput 2017;31(4):677–84.
54. Liu Y, Lou JS, Mi WD, et al. Pulse pressure variation shows a direct linear correlation with tidal volume in anesthetized healthy patients. BMC Anesthesiol 2016; 16:75.

55. Thiele RH, Raghunathan K, Brudney CS, et al. American Society for Enhanced Recovery (ASER) and perioperative quality initiative (POQI) joint consensus statement on perioperative fluid management within an enhanced recovery pathway for colorectal surgery. Perioper Med (Lond) 2016;5:24.
56. Brandstrup B, Svendsen PE, Rasmussen M, et al. Which goal for fluid therapy during colorectal surgery is followed by the best outcome: near-maximal stroke volume or zero fluid balance? Br J Anaesth 2012;109(2):191–9.
57. Abraham-Nordling M, Hjern F, Pollack J, et al. Randomized clinical trial of fluid restriction in colorectal surgery. Br J Surg 2012;99(2):186–91.
58. Wenkui Y, Ning L, Jianfeng G, et al. Restricted peri-operative fluid administration adjusted by serum lactate level improved outcome after major elective surgery for gastrointestinal malignancy. Surgery 2010;147(4):542–52.
59. de Aguilar-Nascimento JE, Diniz BN, do Carmo AV, et al. Clinical benefits after the implementation of a protocol of restricted perioperative intravenous crystalloid fluids in major abdominal operations. World J Surg 2009;33(5):925–30.
60. Joshi GP, Kehlet H. CON: perioperative goal-directed fluid therapy is an essential element of an enhanced recovery protocol? Anesth Analg 2016;122(5):1261–3.
61. Lobo SM, Ronchi LS, Oliveira NE, et al. Restrictive strategy of intraoperative fluid maintenance during optimization of oxygen delivery decreases major complications after high-risk surgery. Crit Care 2011;15(5):R226.
62. Holte K, Sharrock N, Kehlet H. Pathophysiology and clinical implications of perioperative fluid excess. Br J Anaesth 2002;89(4):622–32.
63. Hartmann M, Jonsson K, Zederfeldt B. Effect of tissue perfusion and oxygenation on accumulation of collagen in healing wounds. Randomized study in patients after major abdominal operations. Eur J Surg 1992;158(10):521–6.
64. Kimberger O, Arnberger M, Brandt S, et al. Goal-directed colloid administration improves the microcirculation of healthy and perianastomotic colon. Anesthesiology 2009;110(3):496–504.
65. Cooperman LH, Price HL. Pulmonary edema in the operative and postoperative period: a review of 40 cases. Ann Surg 1970;172(5):883–91.
66. Stein L, Beraud JJ, Cavanilles J, et al. Pulmonary edema during fluid infusion in the absence of heart failure. JAMA 1974;229(1):65–8.
67. Gao T, Li N, Zhang JJ, et al. Restricted intravenous fluid regimen reduces the rate of postoperative complications and alters immunological activity of elderly patients operated for abdominal cancer: a randomized prospective clinical trail. World J Surg 2012;36(5):993–1002.
68. Kawasaki T, Ogata M, Kawasaki C, et al. Effects of epidural anaesthesia on surgical stress-induced immunosuppression during upper abdominal surgery. Br J Anaesth 2007;98:196–203.
69. Utoh J, Yamamoto T, Utsunomiya T, et al. Effect of surgery on neutrophil functions, superoxide and leukotriene production. Br J Surg 1988;75:682–5.
70. Nichols P, Ramsden C, Ward U, et al. Perioperative immunotherapy with recombinant interleukin 2 in patients undergoing surgery for colorectal cancer. Cancer Res 1992;52:5765–9.
71. Kie H, Zhou H, Li Y. Perioperative restricted fluid therapy preserves immunological function in patients with colorectal cancer. World J Gastroenterol 2014; 20(42):15852–9.
72. Kellum J, Song M, Li J. Science review: extracellular acidosis and the immune response: clinical and physiologic implications. Crit Care 2004;8(5):331–6.

73. Kellum JA. Fluid resuscitation and hyperchloremic acidosis in experimental sepsis: improved short-term survival and acid-base balance with Hextend compared with saline. Crit Care Med 2002;30(2):300–5.
74. Holte K. Pathophysiology and clinical implications of peroperative fluid management in elective surgery. Dan Med Bull 2010;57(7):B4156.
75. Fries D, Innerhofer P, Schobersberger W. Time for changing coagulation management in trauma-related massive bleeding. Curr Opin Anaesthesiol 2009;22(2): 267–74.
76. Simmons JW, Powell MF. Acute traumatic coagulopathy: pathophysiology and resuscitation. Br J Anaesth 2016;117(suppl 3):iii31–43.
77. Grocott MP, Mythen MG, Gan TJ. Perioperative fluid management and clinical outcomes in adults. Anesth Analg 2005;100(4):1093–106.
78. Calvert S, Shaw A. Perioperative acute kidney injury. Perioper Med (Lond) 2012; 1(1):6.
79. Goren O, Matot I. Perioperative acute kidney injury. Br J Anaesth 2015; 115(Suppl 2):ii3–14.
80. Cannesson M, Gan TJ. PRO: perioperative goal-directed fluid therapy is an essential element of an enhanced recovery protocol. Anesth Analg 2016; 122(5):1258–60.
81. King MS. Preoperative evaluation. Am Fam Physician 2000;62(2):387–96.

Enhanced Recovery After Surgery

Implementation Strategies, Barriers and Facilitators

Emily A. Pearsall, MSc[a], Robin S. McLeod, MD, FRCSC[b,c],*

KEYWORDS

- Knowledge translation • Implementation • Quality improvement • Barriers
- Facilitators

KEY POINTS

- Assessment of local barriers and enablers before implementation will increase uptake.
- Engagement of all members of the multidisciplinary team is the key to success.
- Collection of baseline data and audit and regular feed back to monitor change is crucial.

INTRODUCTION

Enhanced Recovery after Surgery (ERAS) pathways include several preoperative, intraoperative, and postoperative interventions, which, when implemented together, have been shown to decrease the amount of stress and gut dysfunction in individuals undergoing elective colorectal surgery, and leads to enhanced recovery, decreased morbidity, and length of stay.[1,2] Although each intervention in the ERAS pathway seems to be easy to implement, taken as a whole, ERAS recommendations can be difficult to adopt.[3–7] As shown in **Fig. 1**, ERAS span the patient's entire surgical journey from preadmission to discharge, and during this time, multiple health care providers from different specialties provide care. Thus, without a coordinated approach to care with all care givers working together to ensure that all elements of the ERAS program are implemented and adhered to, the benefits of an ERAS program will not be realized.

There are various implementation frameworks that can be used to implement an ERAS program, including the Institute for Healthcare Improvement (IHI) Model for

---

Disclosure Statement: The authors have nothing to disclose.
[a] Best Practice in Surgery, Department of Surgery, University of Toronto, 149 College Street, 5th Floor, Toronto Ontario M5T 1P5, Canada; [b] Quality and Best Practices, Department of Surgery, University of Toronto, 149 College Street, 5th Floor, Toronto Ontario M5T 1P5, Canada; [c] Clinical Programs and Quality Initiatives, Cancer Care Ontario, 620 University Avenue, 16th floor, Toronto, ON M5G 2L7, Canada
* Corresponding author.
E-mail address: robin.mcleod@cancercare.on.ca

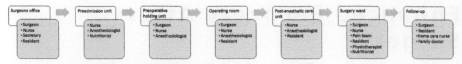

Fig. 1. An ERAS patients' transitions in care.

Improvement,[8] Kotter Eight Step Change Model,[9] Knowledge to Action Cycle (KTA),[10] as well as others. The key components of all of these frameworks are the following:

- The current status should be assessed before implementation
- The quality initiative should be developed based on evidence
- Change management initiatives should be developed to support implementation
- Performance should be measured and feedback provided regularly to all participants

A Cochrane systematic review of 15 studies analyzed whether tailored interventions are more effective than nontailored interventions. The investigators reported a pooled odds ratio of 1.56 (95% confidence interval [CI] 1.27–1.93, $P<.001$) in favor of a tailored intervention and concluded that tailored strategies can be effective but that effect is small to moderate.[11] These results highlight how difficult it is to implement change and multiple strategies are required.

ASSESSMENT OF THE CURRENT STATUS BEFORE IMPLEMENTATION

Collection of baseline data before implementation is essential. Most physicians provide good care to their patients and unless there are data that show that there is a gap in care, they are usually unwilling to make changes. Data are also a powerful tool to assist late adopters in seeing the benefits of ERAS but it is only possible to show an improvement in care if there are baseline data. Furthermore, if possible, baseline data should be collected several months before starting to make changes and educate people on ERAS, because even being aware of the evidence and recommendations may cause a change in practice and then the collected data may not reflect the status at baseline.

Before implementation, potential barriers and facilitators to implementation should also be assessed. This is an essential step in the knowledge to action (KTA) cycle, as Graham and colleagues[10] suggest that implementation strategies will be most effective if they are tailored to each institution's particular set of barriers and enablers. Harrison and colleagues suggest that barriers to implementation may be assessed using known and validated frameworks such as Cabana and colleagues's[12] *Clinical Practice Guidelines Framework for Improvement*, which has been used and modified extensively since its creation in 1999.[13] This framework provides suggestions for questions that may be asked to better understand potential barriers to implementation of new practices. Although it may be useful to follow a specified framework or theoretic model, the essential goal is to determine locally what may hinder implementation. Thus, surveying, interviewing, or even casually speaking to members from all stakeholder groups before implementation might help to understand the local contextual factors.

Several articles have been written specifically about barriers and enablers to the implementation of ERAS programs. Although most studies report both the barriers and facilitators, these factors can often be viewed as both an enabler (if achieved) or a barrier (if missing).

In 2018, Stone and colleagues[14] published a systematic review that included 53 studies to assess the barriers and facilitators to implementation of ERAS programs.

Most were observational studies reporting quantitative data but a third collected qualitative data using surveys or interviews. The *Consolidated Framework for Implementation Research*[15] that consists of 5 domains was used:

1. *Characteristics of the intervention.* The complexity of ERAS guidelines was seen as a barrier due to potentially poor adherence and disruption to the usual surgical practice. Trialability, meaning the ability to pilot the program before widespread implementation, was seen as a potential facilitator. The investigators suggest that adaptability may act both as a facilitator if the intervention is flexible and as a barrier if the intervention has a lack of clear guidance.

2. *Inner setting* refers to factors within the institution. Several barriers and enablers were noted. The creation of networks and having open communication were described as essential strategies to ensure that the multidisciplinary stakeholders communicate and collaborate and create local communities of practice. Leadership engagement was also described as a facilitator because without it, implementation would be difficult to achieve. Institutional resources, including financial resources for structural changes and increased staff, were identified in order to promote early mobilization and eating. In addition, protected time for staff and data collectors was noted as a potential barrier. Compatibility was described as a facilitator when alignment was achieved between ERAS recommendations and the existing culture and also as a barrier when there was inertia to change by physicians and other health care professionals. Lastly, access to the information and having educational materials available to staff and providing educational sessions were assessed as important enablers to implementation.

3. *Outer setting* refers to external factors that might affect implementation. Stone and colleagues identified patient needs and resources as potential barriers if patients had complex comorbidities or there were language barriers or differences in expectations. Working collaboratively with other hospitals as part of the implementation process was also described as a facilitator.

4. The *characteristics of individuals* was largely described as being barriers due to resistance to change by physicians, negative views toward a "cookbook" protocol and lack of support and collaboration among and within disciplines. However, other studies have shown that early adopters and local champions can facilitate implementation and overcome these barriers.[16]

5. The *implementation process* itself was described as a facilitator to implementation. Effective planning involving input from a multidisciplinary team throughout the implementation process was described as important. Similarly, engaging all stakeholders including administrators, front-line staff, and patients and their families in the implementation process is important. The execution of the implementation plan, including the use of formal implementation frameworks with timelines, enables effective implementation. Also, increasing the profile and visibility of ERAS was also considered important in achieving successful implementation. This includes sustaining implementation by consistently providing updates and data back to staff.

In summary, although there are several potential barriers and enablers that affect the implementation of an ERAS program, it is essential to understand which local factors may affect implementation. Before beginning implementation, surveying or interviewing key stakeholders should be performed so implementation strategies can be targeted so what might be barriers can be turned into facilitators.

DEVELOPMENT OF AN ENHANCED RECOVERY AFTER SURGERY PROGRAM BASED ON EVIDENCE

There are multiple meta-analyses showing the benefit of ERAS programs. As well, there are published guidelines that have been developed by institutions and national organizations. These guidelines may vary because there is no established standard and the interventions included in the guidelines may vary as well as the recommendations. As well, some of the recommendations may not have strong evidence supporting them. Although some recommendations may be adopted even though there is no high-level evidence (eg, example early ambulation), generally, if recommendations are not based on moderate-high level evidence, it may be difficult to change practice.

The institution wishing to adopt ERAS may decide to adopt a guideline or alter a guideline to fit the local context. Although the latter will take more effort, the process of reviewing and developing or modifying a guideline is an opportunity to engage all stakeholders, who then assist in the implementation of the recommendations. Either way, sharing the guideline recommendations with all stakeholders before adoption so they can comment on them is important because again, it will increase engagement and ownership of the project.

IMPLEMENTATION STRATEGIES AND CHANGE MANAGEMENT

Several different implementation strategies have been used to implement ERAS programs. Although no studies have evaluated the impact of specific interventions, most studies have reported successful implementation and a change of practice. Of note is that in general, there is limited available evidence on the most effective strategies to implement new evidence into practice. Although there are several methods and theoretical frameworks available for people to choose from, there is little evidence to suggest which ones are most effective. The most commonly reported strategies used to implement ERAS programs are the use of local champions, building communities of practice and multidisciplinary teams, educational meetings, and audit and feedback. In addition to these strategies, patient education and development of standardized materials (orders, pathways etc.) have also been described as useful strategies.[17,18]

Engagement of Stakeholders

Ensuring all stakeholders are aware of ERAS and getting buy-in for its implementation is one of the first actions that should be undertaken. Stakeholders include administration, department heads, surgeons, anesthesiologists, preadmission staff, postanesthetic care unit staff, ward nurses, and other health care professionals including physiotherapists and nutritionists. Ensuring that all stakeholders are aware of the guideline recommendations and the supporting evidence will hopefully increase the uptake of the guideline recommendations especially if the evidence is strong.

Local Champions/Opinion Leaders

Champions refer to local opinion leaders who are often seen as being likable, trustworthy, and influential.[16] In ERAS programs, it is suggested to have champions from surgery, anesthesia, and nursing. The role of a champion is to act as a local point person for their colleagues to go to with questions or concerns and to also act as a liaison with other disciplines and administration. The champions can be nominated, selected, or elected.

Although local champions are felt to be essential, there is little evidence in the scientific literature to support their role in implementation. In 2011, Flodgren and colleagues[16] conducted a systematic review to assess the effectiveness of using local opinion leaders on changing practice and patient outcomes. The review included 18 studies. The investigators found that opinion leaders led to a 12% absolute increase in compliance. When comparing opinion leaders to no intervention, they found a 9% difference in compliance; when compared with a single intervention they found a 14% difference; and when opinion leaders were part of multiintervention compared with no intervention, the investigators found a 10% difference in compliance. They concluded that local opinion leaders, in combination with other interventions or alone, may be a useful strategy to change practice.

The actual activities and roles that the champions undertake are not clearly defined in the literature. Based on their experience, the authors suggest that each hospital should have at least one surgeon, anesthesiologist, and nurse champion.[17]

Multidisciplinary Teams and Communities of Practice

In order for implementation of ERAS programs to succeed, there needs to be buy-in from all disciplines. Most ERAS programs strongly encourage the development of an ERAS implementation team that consists of members from all relevant stakeholder groups, including surgeons, nurses, anesthesiologists, physiotherapists, dieticians, clerks, and hospital administrators as well as residents and other trainees. These teams may be referred to as multidisciplinary, interprofessional, implementation teams or communities of practice. Regardless of their name, the creation of a group of stakeholders to implement ERAS is essential.

The use of communities of practice (CoP) in health care spread from the business sector where they are used to drive knowledge management and as a tool for sharing new knowledge and sharing lessons learned and increasing communication within an organization. Although there is no universal definition of a CoP, there is general consensus that it involves a group of people who share an interest in a topic and want to enhance their knowledge in the area by interacting with others. In 2011, Ranmuthugala and colleagues[19] conducted a systematic review to examine how and why CoPs have been established in health care and whether they are proved to improve practice. They included 31 research papers and 2 systematic reviews. They found no consistency between studies in terms of how the CoPs operate (ie, face to face meetings or online communication) and no information on frequency of meetings. Despite the lack of concrete information on CoPs, there seemed to be a strong interest in determining whether they are effective.

The effect of interprofessional collaboration was studied by Reeves and colleagues[20] in a 2017 Cochrane Review. They included 9 studies that assessed the impact of interventions aimed at increasing interprofessional collaboration. All of the included studies were judged to be of low quality, and thus, the conclusion was that there is insufficient evidence to know the impact of interprofessional collaboration. As well, all of the included studies assessed different activities.

In summary, there seems to be great interest in evaluating the impact of multidisciplinary teams and teamwork in general; however there is little evidence currently available. Despite this, development of local CoPs seems to be strongly recommended for the implementation of ERAS programs.

Educational Meetings

In 2009, Forsetlund and colleagues[21] conducted a Cochrane Review to assess the effects of educational meetings on practice and health care outcomes. In this updated review, 81 trials were included. The investigators found that educational meetings as part of an implementation program compared with no intervention resulted in a 6% increase in compliance with desired practice (interquartile range

[IQR] 1.8–15.9). Educational meetings alone compared with no intervention had a similar effect (risk difference [RD] 6%; IQR 2.9–15.3). On univariate meta-regression analysis, higher attendance was associated with a larger RD ($P<.01$) and mixed interactive and didactic teaching sessions were more effective than didactic teaching sessions (mean adjusted RD 13.6 vs 6.9) or interactive session alone (mean adjusted RD 3.0). The investigators concluded that educational meetings alone or in combination with other interventions may have a small impact on professional practice but less so than other interventions such as audit and feedback.

Patient Education Materials

Many ERAS elements require the active engagement of patients. For example, patients are asked to start mobilizing and eating earlier after surgery. Many ERAS programs created patient education materials to inform patients before surgery about what to expect from their surgery and what is expected of them. Several institutions created their own patient education materials so that they could be tailored to include hospital specific information such as telephone numbers and hospital policies and procedures.

Sibbern and colleagues[22] conducted a systematic review of qualitative studies to synthesize the available information on patient experience within ERAS programs. They included 11 studies. They reported that most patients received written information before a preadmission visit and this information helped them feel prepared for surgery. They also noted that patients often experienced inconsistent messaging between the written and verbal information given to them by health care professionals throughout their surgical journey and this led to increased stress and reduced trust in the caregivers. Patients also expressed mixed feelings toward being active participants in their recovery and feeling motivated and engaged but also felt pressure to recover too quickly. In addition, some patients felt that the ERAS program was too structured and did not allow for individual patient care. Lastly, patients expressed a concern about their readiness for early discharge. Although some patients felt that they were well prepared for an earlier discharge and looked forward to going home sooner, others felt rushed and ill prepared to take care of themselves. Patients' confidence regarding discharge largely depended on the consistency of information provided to them.

Standardized Order Sets

Although there is limited evidence to support the addition of ERAS elements into standardized order sets, there is strong anecdotal evidence to support this. Having the recommendations embedded into standardized care pathways or order sets allows for staff to easily and effectively adhere to recommendations and be reminded of them. It also decreases the chance of new hires, residents, and others who are unfamiliar with ERAS to deviate from the protocol.

Although there is little evidence on the value of standardized orders in ERAS, there is evidence that standardized order sets increase compliance in other areas. The University of Missouri Heath System developed and implemented a standardized order set to improve deep venous thrombosis prophylaxis rates. Two months after implementation, rates increased from 75% to 91% and were sustained at 95% after 1 year.[23] Fleming and colleagues[24] conducted an observational study to examine order set use for evidence-based pneumonia guidelines. The study included 3301 patients and the investigators reported that use of order sets significantly improved compliance (Relative risk (RR) 1.24, 95% CI: 1.04–1.48) and decreased in-hospital mortality (hazard ratio 0.66, 95% CI: 0.45–0.97).

MEASUREMENT AND ASSESSMENT OF PERFORMANCE

Audit and feedback is an essential element in the implementation and maintenance of ERAS. Collecting data and providing regular feedback to stakeholders allows them to know how they are doing and what areas need improvement.

There are some principles for using data to assess performance. Currie and Kennedy suggest that establishing targets is essential.[25] This is important because it may give the team more incentive to reach these targets. As well, feedback should be provided at short intervals (every 6–12 weeks) so the implementation team can implement changes and then determine if they are effective. If not, the team can then consider implementing other strategies to improve uptake. Finally, if audit and feedback is to improve outcome, evidence or guideline recommendations must be available to help the institution to implement a new strategy to improve outcome.

The benefit of audit and feedback was studied by Ivers and colleagues[26] in a Cochrane Review in 2012. They included 140 randomized controlled trials, which attest to the frequency of its use. They found an overall weighted mean absolute increase of 4% (IQR: 1–16) in compliance and also conducted a multivariable analysis that showed that feedback is most effective when baseline data are low, a supervisor or colleague provides the feedback, data are shared more than once and are provided verbally and written, and specific targets and an action plan are in place.

More recently, Tuti and colleagues[27] conducted a systematic review to assess the effectiveness of electronic audit and feedback. They included 9 publications reporting on 7 studies. Benchmarks in the reports often compared individual or local performance to local or national averages. Three studies found a positive effect with electronic audit and feedback on the quality of care, with studies reporting increases in compliance from 9.4% to 14.9% for different interventions. The weighted odds ratio of compliance with desired outcomes was 1.93 (95% CI: 1.36–2.73) when comparing electronic audit and feedback to no audit and feedback. However, because of high heterogeneity, these results may not be reliable.

With regards to ERAS, there are several ways to collect data from simple data collection in an excel spreadsheet to joining a large international database. For example, the European ERAS® Society developed a database specifically to assess the ERAS implementation. One of the benefits of the ERAS® data system is that it is easy to extract data from the database to assess performance because it was developed as a quality improvement tool. One disadvantage, however, is that the variables cannot be changed or modified to suit the individual institutions. Other data collection tools such as the American College of Surgeons National Quality Improvement Program (NSQIP) can be used to assess the implementation of ERAS. NSQIP has a small ERAS data collection subsection that allows individuals to assess their compliance in real-time. Collecting data can be costly especially if there is a dedicated person collecting data. Thus, using existing data collection programs such as NSQIP or creating your own data collection tools using Excel (or something similar) where possible may be preferable. In addition, minimizing the amount of data may also help to minimize the costs.

STRUCTURED ENHANCED RECOVERY AFTER SURGERY IMPLEMENTATION PROGRAMS

The most popular formal ERAS implementation program comes from the European ERAS® Society. The essence of their program is that a structured, multidisciplinary approach is required. In the ERAS® Society program, the creation of ERAS team with members from all involved units as well as having local champions from each specialty and a dedicated ERAS coordinator (nurse or physician assistant) are mandatory.

They strongly recommend consistent weekly meetings to discuss compliance and implement change. Lastly, an essential element of implementation is auditing practice and providing regular feedback.[18] Several institutions have opted to adopt the ERAS® Society implementation program, which includes 3 meetings over the course of a year and a train-the-trainer program. The program involves a medical expert in ERAS and a change management coach trained in ERAS who run the program. Ljungqvist[28] describe in detail their Implementation Program in the SAGES/ERAS® Society Manual. The ERAS® Society created this standardized implementation program based on Breakthrough methodology from the Institute for Healthcare Improvement.

In Canada, a slightly different approach was undertaken in the province of Ontario. Although the strategies were similar, the approach was different. First, the Ontario group, known now as the Best Practice in Surgery, followed the KTA cycle when creating an implementation for ERAS (iERAS) program.[17] The KTA cycle is an iterative process that leads to both the creation and the implementation of new evidence. First, the Best Practice in Surgery created a locally tailored ERAS guideline by systematically reviewing the literature for each known ERAS intervention for colorectal surgery. Several working groups were created to review the evidence and provide recommendations. A local consensus meeting was held with all stakeholders to engage them in the process and to help ensure buy-in for the implementation phase. Before implementation, the group also conducted a retrospective audit of practice at 7 local hospitals to identify current gaps in care.[29] To assess barriers and facilitators, interviews were conducted with nurses, anesthesiologists, and surgeons from 7 local hospitals.[7] As well, residents who were currently rotating through these hospitals were surveyed.[30] These data were then analyzed and used to create a tailored implementation strategy. The implementation strategies included having nurse, surgery, and anesthesia champions at each center who acted as a liaison with the provincial ERAS community of practice and also acted as opinion leaders, educators, and point persons within their hospital. The local champions met locally weekly or biweekly and met with the provincial community of practice via teleconference once a month. Support from hospital administration was also an essential part of the program and hospitals were not able to participate without written support. Standardized order sets and care pathways were developed by participating hospitals before implementation to ensure compliance and sustainability of the program. As well, a patient education booklet and video were created to provide education to all patients before their operation. An ERAS coordinator was an essential part of the program. This role was usually filled by a nurse who prospectively collected data and also assisted with local implementation efforts. Data were collected prospectively and were provided to the sites at 3 monthly intervals. The reports included data from all of the 15 hospitals so hospitals could learn from each other. As well, annual in-person meetings with the champions and other stakeholders from all of the participating centers discuss barriers and enablers to implementation and share lessons learned.

SUMMARY

Implementation of an ERAS program is complex and requires a wide range of change management strategies. As discussed, there are multiple potential barriers and therefore multiple strategies are required to successfully implement it.

After the iERAS program was implemented in the province of Ontario, we learned several lessons. First and foremost, patient and family care givers were not included in the development or implementation of the iERAS program. Although patient education materials were developed, including patients in the planning of the program and getting their guidance on all aspects of the implementation would have been invaluable.

Secondly, ERAS programs should not be considered to be a quality improvement program or project. It should be considered good care for surgical patients, and these recommendations should just be part of the care of the average patient. Despite this nuance, implementing ERAS does require a lot of work, including a culture change. Having patients ambulate on the day of surgery and eat on day 1 are completely against the way patients have been treated for the last 100 years. Leaving catheters in for several days for monitoring and using nasogastric tubes have been engrained in residents. Instead, sending an "ERAS" patient home on postoperative day 3 after major surgery is almost unbelievable! In Ontario we received 2 years of funding to implement the iERAS program. Although we were very successful in many ways, making changes and embedding them in surgical management of patients cannot be done in 2 years. Rather it will likely take 5 to 10 years.

We learned many other things as well: we (1) should have collected baseline data before we started working on the ERAS guideline; (2) collected too much data; (3) should have set targets; and (4) should have improved our communication. Having said that, change can be made and adoption of ERAS programs for all patients, not just patients having colorectal surgery, leads to improved patient care.

REFERENCES

1. Kehlet H, Wilmore DW. Evidence-based surgical care and the evolution of fast-track surgery. Ann Surg 2008;248:189–98.
2. Greco M, Capretti G, Beretta L, et al. Enhanced recovery program in colorectal surgery: a meta-analysis of randomized controlled trials. World J Surg 2014;38:1531–41.
3. Donohoe CL, Nguyen M, Cook J, et al. Fast-track protocols in colorectal surgery. Surgeon 2011;9:95–103.
4. Maessen J, Dejong CH, Hausel J, et al. A protocol is not enough to implement an enhanced recovery programme for colorectal resection. Br J Surg 2007;94:224–31.
5. Gustafsson UO, Hausel J, Thorell A, et al. Adherence to the enhanced recovery after surgery protocol and outcomes after colorectal cancer surgery. Arch Surg 2011;146:571–7.
6. Kahokehr A, Sammour T, Zargar-Shoshtari K, et al. Implementation of ERAS and how to overcome the barriers. Int J Surg 2009;7:16–9.
7. Pearsall EA, Meghji Z, Pitzul KB, et al. A qualitative study to understand the barriers and enablers in implementing an enhanced recovery after surgery program. Ann Surg 2015;261:92–6.
8. Langley GL, Moen R, Nolan KM, et al. The improvement guide: a practical approach to enhancing organizational performance. 2nd edition. San Francisco (CA): Jossey-Bass Publishers; 2009.
9. Kotter JP. Leading change. Boston: Harvard Business School Press; 1996.
10. Graham ID, Logan J, Harrison MB, et al. Lost in knowledge translation: time for a map? J Contin Educ Health Prof 2006;26(1):13–24.
11. Baker R, Camosso-Stefinovic J, Gillies C, et al. Tailored interventions to address determinants of practice. Cochrane Database Syst Rev 2015;(4):CD005470.
12. Cabana MD, Rand CS, Powe NR, et al. Why don't physicians follow clinical practice guidelines? A framework for improvement. JAMA 1999;282(15):1458–65.
13. Harrison MB, Légaré F, Graham ID, et al. Adapting clinical practice guidelines to local context and assessing barriers to their use. CMAJ 2010;182(2):E78–84.
14. Stone AB, Yuan CT, Rosen MA, et al. Barriers to and facilitators of implementing enhanced recovery pathways using an implementation framework: a systematic review. JAMA Surg 2018;153(3):270–9.

15. Damschroder LJ, Aron DC, Keith RE, et al. Fostering implementation of health services research findings into practice: a consolidated framework for advancing implementation science. Implement Sci 2009;4:50.
16. Flodgren G, Parmelli E, Doumit G, et al. Local opinion leaders: effects on professional practice and health care outcomes. Cochrane Database Syst Rev 2011;(8):CD000125.
17. McLeod RS, Aarts MA, Chung F, et al. Development of an enhanced recovery after surgery guideline and implementation strategy based on the knowledge-to-action cycle. Ann Surg 2015;262(6):1016–25.
18. Ljungqvist O, Scott M, Fearon KC. Enhanced recovery after surgery: a review. JAMA Surg 2017;152(3):292–8.
19. Ranmuthugala G, Plumb JJ, Cunningham FC, et al. How and why are communities of practice established in the healthcare sector? A systematic review of the literature. BMC Health Serv Res 2011;11:273.
20. Reeves S, Palaganas J, Zierler B. An updated synthesis of review evidence of interprofessional education. J Allied Health 2017;46(1):56–61.
21. Forsetlund L, Bjørndal A, Rashidian A, et al. Continuing education meetings and workshops: effects on professional practice and health care outcomes. Cochrane Database Syst Rev 2009;(2):CD003030.
22. Sibbern T, Bull Sellevold V, Steindal SA, et al. Patients' experiences of enhanced recovery after surgery: a systematic review of qualitative studies. J Clin Nurs 2017;26(9–10):1172–88.
23. Vyas D, Bearelly D, Boshard B. A multidisciplinary quality improvement educational initiative to improve the rate of deep-vein thrombosis prophylaxis. Int J Pharm Pract 2014;22(1):92–5.
24. Fleming NS, Ogola G, Ballard DJ. Implementing a standardized order set for community-acquired pneumonia: impact on mortality and cost. Jt Comm J Qual Patient Saf 2009;35(8):414–21.
25. Currie A, Kennedy R. Audit: why. In: Feldman L, Delaney C, Ljungqvist O, et al, editors. The SAGES/ERAS® society manual of enhanced recovery programs for gastrointestinal surgery. Basel (Switzerland): Springer; 2015. p. 237–46.
26. Ivers N, Jamtvedt G, Flottorp S, et al. Audit and feedback: effects on professional practice and healthcare outcomes. Cochrane Database Syst Rev 2012;(6):CD000259.
27. Tuti T, Nzinga J, Njoroge M, et al. A systematic review of electronic audit and feedback: intervention effectiveness and use of behaviour change theory. Implement Sci 2017;12(1):61.
28. Ljungqvist O. Introducing enhanced recovery programs into practice: lessons learned from the ERAS® society implementation program. In: Feldman L, Delaney C, Ljungqvist O, et al, editors. The SAGES/ERAS® society manual of enhanced recovery programs for gastrointestinal surgery. Basel (Switzerland): Springer; 2015. p. 215–26.
29. Aarts MA, Okrainec A, Glicksman A, et al. Adoption of enhanced recovery after surgery (ERAS) strategies for colorectal surgery at academic teaching hospitals and impact on total length of hospital stay. Surg Endosc 2012;26(2):442–50.
30. Nadler A, Pearsall EA, Victor JC, et al. Understanding surgical residents' postoperative practices and barriers and enablers to the implementation of an Enhanced Recovery After Surgery (ERAS) Guideline. J Surg Educ 2014;71(4):632–8.

Nursing Perspectives on Enhanced Recovery After Surgery

Daran Brown, MBA, RN[a],*, Anisa Xhaja, MHA, MSHQS[b]

KEYWORDS

- Nursing barriers • Enhanced recovery after surgery • ERAS • ERAS nursing

KEY POINTS

- Nursing leadership and buy-in are important in a successful enhanced recovery after surgery (ERAS) implementation.
- Standardized ERAS nursing staff education improves compliance with nursing-specific ERAS measures.
- Overcoming key nursing barriers improves ERAS pathway compliance.
- Hospital-wide implementation of ERAS clinical pathways can be done through the introduction of a centralized project management structure.

A growing body of evidence suggests that the implementation of an Enhanced Recovery After Surgery (ERAS) clinical pathway can accelerate recovery and reduce length of stay for patients undergoing major surgery through multimodal strategies, such as optimal pain relief, stress reduction, early nutrition, and early mobilization.[1] Further evidence suggests compliance with all the ERAS elements drives its effectiveness.[1] Adherence to all individual elements, however, is difficult. In an international multicenter study, compliance with individual ERAS processes varied significantly from 13% to 100%.[2] Further studies demonstrate that adherence rates to ERAS guidelines are particularly low in the postoperative care with fewer than half of patients reporting completion of some aspect of their planned postoperative care regimen.[3] The majority of available research about ERAS implementation has focused on the perspective and impact of the role of the surgeon. Given the interdisciplinary nature of patient care, however, other care team members, such as nurses, hold the key to overcome ERAS implementation barriers and compliance to ERAS processes.[2] The successful implementation of ERAS relies heavily on the daily patient care that nursing staff leads throughout the continuum of care.[4] Although ERAS, as a clinical pathway, provides an

Disclosure Statement: The authors have nothing to disclose.
[a] Department of Quality and Patient Safety, UAB Hospital, 619 19th Street South JT1450, Birmingham, AL 35249, USA; [b] Quality, Patient Safety and Clinical Effectiveness, UAB Hospital, 619 19th Street South JT1402, Birmingham, AL 35249, USA
* Corresponding author.
E-mail address: daranbrown@uabmc.edu

interdisciplinary approach to care delivery, nurses are in the forefront of that care delivery, carrying out daily tasks and assuring compliance with ERAS pathway elements. Understanding the role that nursing holds in ERAS pathway implementation remains an area for further research. This article explores the role nursing plays in the implementation of an ERAS pathway in an academic medical center. It further describes the key barriers (**Table 1**) faced by nursing staff and how overcoming these barriers is critical to a successful ERAS program.

ADAPTATION OF EVIDENCE-BASED PRACTICE

Behavior change is difficult in any industry and implementing change in health care is no different. Although the evidence-based ERAS pathway has improved patient care, its adaptation in the United States has been slow due to a variety of challenges: organizational culture, lack of resources, limited time, and buy-in from providers and nursing staff.[5] These challenges are not limited to the implementation of ERAS but rather to all evidence-based approaches because they fundamentally challenge organizational mindset of "that's the way we have always done it." This challenge was observed initially in nurse clinicians' acceptance of ERAS pathway. ERAS, unlike any other pathway, redefines the surgical preparation and management of patients from the outpatient setting in the clinic consultation to discharge. This phenomenon was demonstrated in a descriptive study of Melnyk and colleagues[6] at Ohio State University, in which only 34.5% of the participants "agreed" or "strongly agreed" that they consistently used evidence-based practice (EBP) in treating their patients. The Institute of Medicine 2020 goal of clinical decision making being evidence-based is 90%.[6] Therefore, nurse leaders and educators have considerable opportunity to narrow this gap and establish an organizational nursing culture where EBP is supported and adopted.

McLeod and colleagues[7] described several universal barriers, to all health disciplines, in the implementation of ERAS, including lack of work force, lack of hospital resources, lack of buy-in, and poor communication among team members. Discipline-specific issues were identified; most nurses believed that early feeding was not important and that workforce issues were barriers to early ambulation.[7] Similar findings were observed at the authors' institution, where the compliance and the support of ERAS as an EBP in the initial grassroots efforts by nursing was initially resisted. This resistance and hesitation were due to several reasons: (1) ERAS challenged existing practice, (2) turnover in nursing leadership, (3) high nursing staff turnover and high nursing burnout, and (4) lack of consistent nursing educators, education content, and plan.

ERAS was one of several hospital priorities among other hospital priorities for example, throughput, sepsis, bar code scanning just to mention a few, for the nurse managers and frontline nursing staff in the beginning stages of implementation. It was a new way of thinking and providing care for their surgical patients; one that contradicted some older practices, such as not allowing an immediate postoperative diet and not allowing immediate postoperative mobilization. There was not a unified buy-in from nursing leaders from the 4 main clinical areas involved in the surgical patient care pathway: clinic, preoperative holding, operating room, postanesthesia care unit, and nursing floors. Many of them had historically worked in silos, meaning quality improvement projects were done exclusively in their respective areas without communicating and considering their impact downstream or upstream throughout the continuum of care. As a result, it was difficult to break those silos to educate, implement, and sustain ERAS processes in each area.

Henderson and Fletcher[8] described that nursing staff's view on EPB was passive and that they saw it as tick-box exercise and non–value added, which led to

Table 1
Summary of nursing barriers in an effective enhanced recovery after surgery program implementation

Nursing Barriers	Subcategories	Mitigation Strategies	Responsible Parties
Adoption of EBPs	ERAS is an EBPs	1. Integrate ERAS implementation as an annual strategic goal and align it appropriately with the additional nursing goals	Chief nursing officer, Nursing directors, Nursing managers
Nursing staffing	Leadership turnover	1. Create a culture of safety 2. Manage nursing leadership priorities and include time dedicated to ERAS implementation 3. Reward high performers	Chief nursing officer, Nursing directors
	Frontline staff turnover	1. Create a culture of safety 2. Manage the projects that frontline nurses are undertaking 3. Educate the "why" behind ERAS implementation 4. Reward high performers	Nursing manager, Nursing educators
	Culture and behaviors	1. Obtain buy-in for ERAS at the hospital and nursing leadership level (ie, chief nursing officer, chief executive officer, and assistant vice presidents) 2. Support nursing leadership with time to dedicate to new EBP initiatives such as ERAS	Chief nursing officer, Nursing directors, Nursing managers
	Education	1. Create a consistent ERAS education pathway for nurses 2. Create education plan for new and existing nursing staff	Nursing manager, Nursing educators
Hospital resources	ERAS coordinator	1. Create a business case for the role and its importance in patient outcomes to include return on investment	ERAS coordinator, Project manager, Hospital leadership
	Wound ostomy nurses	1. Assess needs of organization	ERAS coordinator
	Data availability	1. Creating a role that oversees data 2. Build ERAS-specific dashboards 3. Publish ERAS process metrics 4. Conduct weekly manual chart audits (first 8 wk of implementation) 5. Publish monthly data updates 6. Encourage organizational transparency in data sharing	Nursing leadership, Nursing educator

frustrations. For example, in the authors' institution, patient education in the clinic was not done consistently nor was it documented in the electronic medical records. Nurses in the clinic had many tasks and were seeing a large number of patients. Spending 5 minutes to 10 minutes to educate their patients about ERAS, with facilitated use of the teach-back method, was seen by nursing staff as extra work. Furthermore, documentation of the education in the electronic medical record was seen as unnecessary extra clicks. Meanwhile, patients and their families want to be involved proactively about their surgery pathway and prepare for what they should expect.[9] Therefore, education preoperatively is important.

Early mobilization was another challenge faced by nursing staff, although there were several studies demonstrating its safety.[10] This was similar in the authors' organization, where frontline nurses feared that early patient mobilization on the day of surgery would increase the unit's fall rates and hurt the patients. They simply were not comfortable with moving their patients and saw patient mobilization as a physical therapy function and not one for nursing.

Medical, nursing, and allied health staff acknowledged difficulties in changing behavior. This was particularly apparent for the more experienced staff for whom change in practice was identified as more difficult.[2] Patients were historically placed on liquid diets postsurgery pre-ERAS. As a result, many nurses from the authors' colorectal surgical postoperative unit believed that allowing patients to resume a regular diet on postoperative day 0 led patients to make poor nutritional choices, resulting in increased nausea and vomiting the days after the surgery. This challenge eased over time, although a view persisted that ERAS care pathway required some individualization.

Initiation of any evidenced-based practice, such as an ERAS clinical pathway implementation, can place pressure on nursing staff. The time constraints of patient care have been identified as a primary challenge in integrating EBP into nursing practice.[8] At the authors' institution, this concern was evident in the early stages of ERAS implementation, with nurses verbalizing a fear of an increased workload, including additional charting requirements. The nursing staff believed that it was the responsibility of nursing management to provide them with tools that aided staff in providing patient education in a more efficient manner. Requests were made by the staff to provide specific materials, such as informational handouts, that reinforced ERAS education and knowledge. It was believed that these materials would aid the nursing staff in making more efficient use of their time. This may explain why nurses, in the study performed by Henderson and Fletcher,[8] viewed access to EBP as passive in nature, with nurses expecting that management provide staff with evidence-based tools and policies to aid in nursing practice.[8] The specific tools developed and used at the authors' institution have included nutritional guides, handouts on management of pain, and an ostomy booklet tracking guide for patients. Importantly, all tools were suggested by the nursing staff to aid them in time management while reinforcing patient education.

NURSING LEADERSHIP

Nursing leadership is paramount in the buy-in and adaptation of EBPs. This is integral in not only teaching the frontline staff the importance of EBP but also, most importantly, incorporating it in day-to-day work and patient care. The consistency of information sharing of EBP to nursing work force in each clinical area is important in the adaptation of ERAS across the continuum. The nursing champion of the ERAS colorectal surgery project managed the postoperative care unit in the authors' institution and was only able to implement the postoperative ERAS elements in the colorectal surgical postoperative nursing unit. He did not have control over or authority in other nursing-based clinical areas (clinic and perioperative areas). Therefore, the compliance of preoperative ERAS elements, such as ERAS patient education documentation in the clinic, was low, at maximum 37%. Identification of respected champions who provide peer education and encourage interprofessional communication and collaboration was cited as an enabler to increase the likelihood of adoption of an ERAS protocol.[7] The authors' institution's low patient education documentation rates in the preoperative clinic may demonstrate the effect of not having an ERAS champion in place providing daily education and encouragement to the preoperative clinical staff.

Successful change management and ERAS implementation occur as a process that evolves from leadership, creation of the climate for change, and engagement and empowerment of those involved, through the development of a change initiative, implementation, or trial of the pathway and sustained change with continued improvement.[11] Furthermore, a supportive nurse manager who is a good leader is instrumental in creating the nurse practice environment needed to achieve quality patient outcomes.[12] One nurse manager from 1 clinical area, however, needs the nursing leadership support to take a large initiative, such as ERAS, which touches many clinical areas across the continuum of care. Therefore, the initial grassroots effort to implement ERAS in different clinical areas led by a single nurse champion, who was located in the postoperative nursing unit, was limited because the executive nursing leadership had not bought into the benefits of the ERAS process. Executive nursing leaders sought improved patient outcomes before providing additional resources to the ERAS implementation across the continuum of care.

The dissemination of ERAS to other surgical service lines depends on the leadership, and organizations are taking different approaches to developing a systematic framework to implement ERAS effectively and efficiently across hospitals and health systems. The Alberta Health Services in Canada used the 6-step Quality Enhancement Research Initiative model to implement and monitor end-to-end ERAS implementation that included identifying the high-risk surgical areas, defining their respective best practices from the ERAS® Society, outlining existing processes, implementing best practice interventions, and recording the improved outcomes and those that improved patients' health overall.[13] They began initially in 2 sites and after 9 months to 12 months expanded to 4 additional sites[13] The Alberta Health Services used another tool, the Theoretical Domains Framework, to approach change in behavior through a simple 4-step process: identifying who needs change, identifying what barriers need to be addressed, identifying the interventions, and measuring the change in behavior.[13] This structured, systematic approach of disseminating ERAS throughout 6 Alberta hospitals was successful because it helped leadership start at a smaller scale in 2 hospitals initially, learn and gain insight from those early efforts, and improve the spread and scale of ERAS implementation throughout the health system by providing clear steps and guidelines for their leadership to follow.

The leadership in the authors' organization followed a less structured approach and on a much smaller scale than the Alberta Health Services. The approach was to implement ERAS on 1 surgical service line at a time, allowing that respective surgical leadership to make the case for future implementation of ERAS outside of that service line. Almost 2 years from the first colorectal surgery patient using the ERAS clinical pathway, the ERAS gynecologic oncology clinical pathway was launched. Unlike colorectal surgery, the nursing staff from the clinic to discharge embraced ERAS as a new EBP because they saw the improved patient outcomes in the colorectal surgical patients. In addition, 2 years later, there was institutional awareness about ERAS and its results in improving patient outcomes and patient experience. As such, the

ERAS clinical pathway was supported by the chief nursing officer and the perioperative nursing vice president and was made a priority among the different clinical disciplines involved. The adaptation of EBPs is easier when outcomes are seen firsthand and there are data available to support them. In this case, having the nursing and administrative leadership support, the gynecologic oncology department jumped on the opportunity and successfully and effectively implement ERAS in their patient population in a 3-month period versus the colorectal surgery ERAS implementation (6 months).

NURSING TURNOVER

Nursing staff is integral to implementing change and redesigning health care delivery.[14] More importantly it is the consistency of staff and low nursing turnovers that allow for a stable environment where new EBP can be adopted and sustained. A summary review of nursing turnover research studied the financial and quality impact of high nursing turnover rates to health care organizations.[15] Aside from a high direct cost of recruiting and hiring nurses, nursing turnover is stressful for the remaining staff who has to adjust to the newer nurses coming on board.[16] As nursing staff turnover increases, communication among nursing teams is disrupted, consensus decreases, employee satisfaction is reduced, and in turn nurses who had no intent of changing roles begin to leave due to the high stress, lack of cohesiveness, higher work load, and overall decreased morale.[15] Nursing turnover begins with a stable nurse manager. Nurse managers are among the most important leaders who can create healthy nurse work environments and in turn stable nursing workforces that can improve the quality of patient outcomes.[12] Therefore, it is paramount that health care organizations take the necessary steps to improve retention of experienced nurse leaders. It is the nurse leaders who drive change in an organization and help sustain success. As discussed previously, nursing staff plays a key role in transforming nursing practices, but a key barrier to a successful health care transformation is the high nursing staff turnover.[14]

One of the main barriers observed during the early implementation of ERAS pathway at the authors' organization's colorectal surgery was the departure of the nurse manager and nurse educator of the postoperative colorectal surgical nursing unit. This initial departure led the inpatient surgery nursing unit to have 3 different nurse managers during a 3-year span. In addition, it had 2 different nurse educators during that same time period. The change in nursing leadership and unit nurse educator resulted in gaps of education for the frontline nursing staff regarding ERAS, its processes, its importance to patient care, and patient care outcomes. Each new nurse manager and nurse educator started from the beginning in terms of learning about ERAS and adopting it in their daily work. They, themselves, had a steep learning curve to overcome before they could be a resource to their nursing staff. New management had to learn the ERAS process in the clinic and perioperative care settings before disseminating it into their nursing teams. This made it difficult to sustain and improve compliance with ERAS elements on the colorectal surgical postoperative nursing unit in the initial stages of ERAS implementation.

One of the main differences between the initial ERAS colorectal surgery implementation and the more recent ERAS gynecologic oncology implementation was the absence of turnover in the gynecologic oncology postoperative nursing unit leadership. The gynecologic oncology unit had one consistent nurse manager and one nurse educator throughout the design, education, and implementation of ERAS pathway. This provided consistent leadership and accountability in meeting designed ERAS processes that was lacking in the colorectal surgery group due to their nursing leadership turnover.

In addition, nursing leaders from the clinic; preoperative assessment, consultation, and treatment; preoperative holding; operating room; and postanesthesia care unit were present and engaged throughout the design of the ERAS gynecologic oncology pathway development, facilitating the decision making and troubleshooting any barriers. They observed firsthand the colorectal surgery ERAS patients in their clinical areas and the positive change it brought to not only the patients but also to the nursing staff.

Nursing turnover is present in many health care organizations related to an identified national nursing shortage, which leads to possible staff satisfaction issues. Organizations implementing new and innovative clinical pathways, such as ERAS, need to pay close attention to retention strategies of not only frontline nursing staff but also nursing leaders to support, disseminate, and sustain existing and future quality improvement efforts in their respective organizations.

NURSING STAFF EDUCATION

Patient safety is now a national imperative, and health care organizations must use initiatives that reliably produce the safest environments. In turn, clinicians must be knowledgeable about the evidence that demonstrates these expected safety outcomes.[16] Specifically, education and training of nursing staff play an essential role in improving the quality of patient care.[17] Aiken and colleagues[18] demonstrated that nursing education, specifically the effect of increasing bachelor of science nurses by 10% in 665 hospitals in 4 large states, decreased the 30-day inpatient mortality and failure-to-rescue by approximately 4%. Staff education in today's fast-paced health care environment is important in keeping up-to-date with all the new literature and EBPs while assuring their appropriate adoption. Similarly, a coordinated education plan of new care pathway, such as ERAS clinical pathway implementation, is essential in its success and sustainment throughout the continuum of patient care.[4]

The early ERAS staff education for the colorectal surgical pathway in the authors' organization was fragmented and inconsistent. Each clinical area leader developed respective staff education and conducted the education as deemed appropriate, depending on respective staff and working shifts. There was no cohesive education plan or education material to assure that the message was consistent throughout the different nursing clinical care areas, from the ambulatory areas to discharge. The method of education also varied. Some areas held in-person education sessions, some included it in their daily huddles, and some sent out e-mails and posted posters in the staff rooms. Because the ERAS colorectal surgery was the first ERAS pathway implemented, there were many changes that happened along the design phase and implementation as the team found better ways to set up the different ERAS process and tweak them. The lack of a joint, comprehensive, and coordinated staff education and communication resulted in gaps in education, variation in the care provided, and lower compliance with ERAS processes. In addition, due to the decentralized nursing staff education, there was no assurance that all nursing staff, from the ambulatory clinical areas through discharge, received the same education material and understood the "why" behind ERAS and how their ERAS responsibilities may affect other care areas along the continuum of care.

The nursing staff education in the later implementation of ERAS, such as in the ERAS gynecologic oncology pathway, was more organized and structured. One month was dedicated to all staff education to include nurses, patient care technicians, anesthesiology faculty, anesthesiology residents and fellows, surgical faculty, surgery residents, and fellows from all the clinical areas where an ERAS patient received care. The same message was communicated throughout, and all the nurses from the different care areas learned about the entire ERAS pathway from the clinic to discharge. In addition, the nurse educator in the gynecologic oncology postoperative surgery unit created a centralized ERAS folder and engaged the nursing staff in creating it, thus creating a sense of ownership in the process from the frontline nurses. Several education sessions were held for the clinic and floor nurses to attend. Those sessions were led by the lead surgeon which created a sense of a unified and team effort in implementing ERAS but also leading to its success in the gynecologic surgical patient population. This method of nursing education was well received by frontline nursing staff and proved helpful in a greater buy-in by nursing of this new care pathway. In addition, the availability of internal data from the ERAS colorectal surgery group helped boost their confidence in the process.

RESOURCE AND PROCESS LIMITATIONS
Centralized Project Management

Lyon and colleagues[2] found that staff participants in an ERAS program found that an ERAS coordinator improved availability for patient education and staff ability to follow the ERAS protocol. One of the main barriers to implementing an effective ERAS program as described in the study fell in the category of "Health system resources," specifically the role of an ERAS coordinator.[2] All study participants viewed the ERAS coordinator as a vital link to ERAS implementation because this position would be responsible for auditing and ensuring that all clinical disciplines among all clinical areas followed the protocol.[2]

An ERAS coordinator position was not explored during the early ERAS implementation at the authors' organization. The early efforts of implementing the ERAS colorectal surgery pathway were led by 2 busy providers and a busy nurse manager. One of the main limitations was lack of institutional support with a centralized project manager function to manage and lead the different phases of design, education, and implementation of the ERAS clinical pathway. This was a barrier of expanding ERAS program beyond the initial surgeon who introduced the institution to the ERAS clinical pathway. Approximately 40 patients underwent ERAS in the first 6 months of ERAS colorectal surgery implementation. The patients were followed by the 2 providers and the nurse manager. One surgery resident tracked compliance of the ERAS elements in an Excel spreadsheet by reviewing each ERAS patient's chart. The team lacked a standardized ERAS patient education booklet; standardized ERAS order sets to guide the care on the inpatient surgical postoperative nursing unit; and an electronic method of identification and communication of ERAS patients along the care continuum. In addition, there were no real-time data available to share with the implementation team.

Approximately 6 months after initiation of the grassroots efforts in the ERAS colorectal surgical patients, a dedicated project manager and a quality improvement nurse were assigned to expand and operationalize the ERAS colorectal surgery pathway and further lead the implementation of ERAS clinical pathway in several key surgical services, such as urology, gynecologic oncology, and obstetrics. ERAS was seen as an optimal surgical pathway by many of the surgical services, gaining institutional support from the administrative and the clinical leaders of the organization. The institutional support of a project management infrastructure alleviated several of the nursing barriers that the grassroots colorectal surgery team encountered in the early stages of ERAS implementation. The dedicated resources made possible a quicker and more effective implementation of ERAS. In addition, the centralized project management facilitated the hard wiring of the new processes put in place as part of the

ERAS clinical pathways in all clinical care areas involved through the development of shared centralized ERAS dashboard accessible to anyone in the organization.

The project management infrastructure was also crucial in creating and disseminating a coordinated and comprehensive education to all clinical and nonclinical staff involved throughout the continuum of care. As such, a sense of responsibility and accountability was planted throughout as each clinical discipline realized that each had an important role in caring for the patient throughout the ERAS pathway.

Wound Ostomy Nurses

The relationship of nurse-trained stoma specialists who can educate and counsel patients on care and potentially reduce stoma-related complications remains an area for ongoing study. A recent study has shown that preoperative and postoperative stoma education in an enhanced recovery program is associated with a significantly shorter hospital stay without any difference in readmission rate or early stoma-related complications[19] Yet, the study by Lyon and colleagues[2] noted that absence of stoma therapy on the weekend hindered earlier discharge of patients because the patients who had surgeries on Fridays missed 2 stoma therapy sessions and 2 educational opportunities during the weekend. Similarly, the limited availability of wound ostomy therapy nurses during the weekend at the authors' organization was a barrier to appropriate and timely education of patients and their timely discharge. A delay in care was observed for those patients whose surgery was in that later part of the week. The first ERAS cohort in colorectal surgery brought to light the need for more wound ostomy nurses within the organization. As a result, the hospital clinical and administrative leaders supported the expansion of the wound ostomy nursing team from 4 nurses to 9 nurses to meet all the needs in the ERAS pathways that followed.

Real-Time Data Availability and Compliance

Good surgical practice is based on ongoing audits of clinical outcomes. It is essential that outcomes be documented during the introduction of an enhanced recovery program1. Auditing the compliance with ERAS processes poses multiple challenges. One study on adherence rates of 13 multimodal measures, included in a colorectal surgery ERAS program, showed that on average only 7.4 of the measures were complied with on a case-by-case basis.[20] This variability in compliance to ERAS measures reflects the complexity and interdisciplinary nature of colorectal surgical care, which is likely to involve staff from multiple disciplines with their respective responsibilities in carrying out portions of a patient's care. As a result, confusion is created across the multidisciplinary team on whose responsibility it is to carry out a certain ERAS measure and document it in the electronic medical records. For example, in the ERAS colorectal surgery pathway implementation, 3 disciplines, including nursing, patient care technicians, and physical therapists, have the responsibility to mobilize ERAS patients on postoperative day 0. Each of them was also responsible for documentation of the mobility of the patient in the electronic medical record. In the initial grassroots launch of ERAS in the colorectal surgery population, focus was placed on ensuring early mobilization occurred. Little focus was placed, however, on educating nursing staff of the importance of documenting mobilization in the electronic medical record.

Furthermore, robust auditing on charted metrics was not an area of focus initially because the data were not readily available to the nurse leader and to the implementation team. No metrics or reports were built to measure the process and the staff compliance with the ERAS elements. The compliance was done by chart audits but the data were not readily available to the implementation team. As a result, it was difficult for the projects nurse leader of the postoperative surgery colorectal surgery nursing unit to audit compliance and hard wire the ERAS processes with the nursing staff.

After onset of the institutional project management, however, support nursing management was provided with compliance reports on nursing-driven ERAS metrics, a marked increase in mobility compliance was identified. Real-time data were made available as ERAS-specific process metrics were built and ERAS-specific dashboards were created for each ERAS clinical pathway implemented. The ERAS gynecologic oncology team had access to electronically driven biweekly and monthly ERAS data. The biweekly data were done through auditing patient charts and communicating the performance with the interdisciplinary ERAS implementation team. Each team lead reviewed data and communicated it to the respective frontline nursing staff for encouragement and improvement purposes. This access of data proved successful in addressing real-time areas of opportunities and providing solutions to nursing staff. In addition, the gynecologic oncology department hired a quality administrator whose role, among other responsibilities, was to oversee the compliance of ERAS process for the ERAS gynecologic oncology pathway to sustain the project long term. The ERAS colorectal surgery pathway did not have such administrative support during the grassroots launch, which hindered the efforts of creating a robust data reporting structure.

SUMMARY

ERAS pathways can achieve better patient recovery. Although their clinical effectiveness depends on many factors, nursing staff and leaders are crucial to the success of an ERAS program. Each project implementation cycle should embrace a multidisciplinary approach with involvement of frontline staff—troops on the ground—as being essential. Nursing barriers to ERAS also exist but may be overcome through support from institutional leadership and empowerment of nurses with consistent education, resources, and communication.

Nursing plays an indispensable role in the adoption, dissemination, and sustainment of an ERAS clinical pathway and an ERAS program within a health care organization or culture. As such, dedicated efforts must be taken by clinical and administrative health care leaders to secure the appropriate support in overcoming the barriers outlined in this article and effectively adopt ERAS throughout.

REFERENCES

1. Fearon KC, Ljungqvist O, Von Meyenfeldt M, et al. Enhanced recovery after surgery: a consensus review of clinical care for patients undergoing colonic resection. Clin Nutr 2005;24(3):466–77.
2. Lyon A, Solomon MJ, Harrison JD. A qualitative study assessing the barriers to implementation of enhanced recovery after surgery. World J Surg 2014;38(6): 1374–80.
3. Kahokehr A, Sammour T, Zargar-Shoshtari K, et al. Implementation of ERAS and how to overcome the barriers. Int J Surg 2009;7(1):16–9.
4. Bryan S, Dukes S. The enhanced recovery programme for stoma patients: an audit. Br J Nurs 2010;19(13):831–4.
5. Gotlib Conn L, McKenzie M, Pearsall EA, et al. Successful implementation of an enhanced recovery after surgery programme for elective colorectal surgery: a process evaluation of champions' experiences. Implementation Sci 2015;10:99.
6. Melnyk BM, Fineout-Overholt E, Gallagher-Ford L, et al. The state of evidence-based practice in US nurses: critical implications for nurse leaders and educators. J Nurs Adm 2012;42(9):410–7.

7. McLeod RS, Aarts MA, Chung F, et al. Development of an enhanced recovery after surgery guideline and implementation strategy based on the knowledge-to-action cycle. Ann Surg 2015;262(6):1016–25.
8. Henderson EM, Fletcher M. Nursing culture: an enemy of evidence-based practice? A focus group exploration. J Child Health Care 2015;19(4):550–7.
9. Poland F, Spalding N, Gregory S, et al. Developing patient education to enhance recovery after colorectal surgery through action research: a qualitative study. BMJ Open 2017;7(6):e013498.
10. de Groot JJ, van Es LE, Maessen JM, et al. Diffusion of enhanced recovery principles in gynecologic oncology surgery: is active implementation still necessary? Gynecol Oncol 2014;134(3):570–5.
11. Anesthetists AAoN. Enhanced recovery after surgery. 2018. Available at: https://www.aana.com/practice/clinical-practice-resources/enhanced-recovery-after-surgery. Accessed April 25, 2018.
12. Warshawsky N, Rayens MK, Stefaniak K, et al. The effect of nurse manager turnover on patient fall and pressure ulcer rates. J Nurs Manag 2013;21(5):725–32.
13. Gramlich LM, Sheppard CE, Wasylak T, et al. Implementation of enhanced recovery after surgery: a strategy to transform surgical care across a health system. Implementation Sci 2017;12(1):67.
14. Kunic RJ, Jackson D. Transforming nursing practice: barriers and solutions. AORN J 2013;98(3):235–48.
15. Tai TW, Bame SI, Robinson CD. Review of nursing turnover research, 1977-1996. Social Sci Med 1998;47(12):1905–24.
16. Balakas K, Sparks L, Steurer L, et al. An outcome of evidence-based practice education: sustained clinical decision-making among bedside nurses. J Pediatr Nurs 2013;28(5):479–85.
17. Chaghari M, Saffari M, Ebadi A, et al. Empowering education: a new model for in-service training of nursing staff. J Adv Med Educ Prof 2017;5(1):26–32.
18. Aiken LH, Cimiotti JP, Sloane DM, et al. Effects of nurse staffing and nurse education on patient deaths in hospitals with different nurse work environments. The J Nurs Adm 2012;42(10 Suppl):S10–6.
19. Forsmo HM, Pfeffer F, Rasdal A, et al. Pre- and postoperative stoma education and guidance within an enhanced recovery after surgery (ERAS) programme reduces length of hospital stay in colorectal surgery. Int J Surg (London, England) 2016;36(Pt A):121–6.
20. Polle SW, Wind J, Fuhring JW, et al. Implementation of a fast-track perioperative care program: what are the difficulties? Dig Surg 2007;24(6):441–9.

Enhanced Recovery After Surgery and Surgical Disparities

Isabel C. Marques, MD, Tyler S. Wahl, MD, MSPH,
Daniel I. Chu, MD*

KEYWORDS

- ERAS • Surgical disparities • Health disparities • Surgical outcomes • Interventions

KEY POINTS

- Health disparities exist in surgery, and they arise from patient, provider and health care system factors.
- Certain surgical populations experience disproportionately worse outcomes, including prolonged postoperative lengths of stay, and higher risks for readmissions.
- Enhanced Recovery After Surgery (ERAS) delivers best-evidence surgical care to all patients through a systematic approach.
- ERAS programs offer a pragmatic and patient-centered way to eliminate disparities and achieve equitable surgical care.

INTRODUCTION

Enhanced Recovery After Surgery (ERAS) pathways use standardized, multimodal perioperative strategies to reduce the physiologic stress and organ dysfunction induced by surgery. Through the systematic delivery of 15 to 20 best-evidence care processes across the entire perioperative spectrum, ERAS achieves earlier recovery after surgery. These evidence-supported processes include, but are not limited to, patient education, multimodal analgesia, fluid optimization, early nutrition, and early mobility.[1] Over the past 2 decades, ERAS has been consistently shown to reduce perioperative morbidity with shorter postoperative lengths of stay and fewer postoperative complications without increasing readmission or mortality rates.[2–7] The benefits to patients, providers, and health care systems are clear across many surgical disciplines, but less is understood about its effects on vulnerable surgical populations.

In 2002, the Institute of Medicine's report, "Unequal Treatment: Confronting Racial and Ethnic Disparities in Healthcare," highlighted the burdens of health-related

Disclosure Statement: The authors have nothing to disclose.
Department of Surgery, University of Alabama at Birmingham, Birmingham, AL, USA
* Corresponding author. Department of Surgery, University of Alabama at Birmingham, 1720 2nd Avenue South Kracke Building 427, Birmingham, AL 35294-0016.
E-mail address: dchu@uabmc.edu

disparities to the health care system. In this report, health disparities were defined as "differences in the quality of health care that are not due to access-related factors or clinical needs, preferences or appropriateness of intervention."[8] This definition has continued to evolve. In Healthy People 2020, the US Department of Health and Human Services (DHHS) defined health-related disparities as "a particular type of health difference that is closely linked with social, economic, and/or environmental disadvantage."[9] The Centers for Disease Control and Prevention further characterized health disparities as a multifaceted and multidisciplinary public health problem.[10] Although most studies to date have focused on health disparities in chronic medical conditions, the significance of disparities in the surgical field has been recently recognized. In 2015, the National Institutes of Health (NIH) and the American College of Surgeons (ACS) convened to develop strategies to address surgical disparities. In a joint statement, the NIH/ACS announced a call to action with a comprehensive research agenda and created new opportunities to support research, including R01 and R21 funding mechanisms.[11] These developments are quite significant and will accelerate national efforts to identify, understand, and eliminate surgical disparities.

THE SCOPE OF SURGICAL DISPARITIES

Up to 30% of the global burden of disease requires surgical care.[12] With these increasing surgical encounters come the associated, and costly, risks of postoperative morbidity and mortality.[12,13] Among surgical populations, it is increasingly clear that certain groups, such as racial/ethnic minorities like African Americans, suffer from worse surgical outcomes compared with other groups.[4,8] These racial/ethnic disparities exist in almost all surgical disciplines, including colorectal,[14] cardiac,[15] oncologic,[16,17] urologic,[18] trauma,[19] and orthopedic[20] surgery. In **Fig. 1**, we show a word

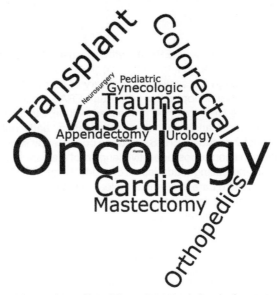

Fig. 1. Surgical specialties where disparities exist. Word cloud of recent systemic review of surgical disparities with updates. PubMed search with keywords: "healthcare disparities" AND "surgery" AND "outcome" AND "US." Size of font reflects the number of publication on the field. (*Data from* Haider AH, Scott VK, Rehman KA, et al. Racial disparities in surgical care and outcomes in the United States: a comprehensive review of patient, provider, and systemic factors. J Am Coll Surg 2013;216(3):482–92.e12.)

cloud summarizing the distribution of surgical disparities research by specialty using results from a previous systematic review[21] and an updated search on the electronic database PubMed (search criteria: "healthcare disparities" AND "surgery" AND "outcome" AND "US" between September 2003 and February 2018). Although the exact burden of surgical disparities is unknown, the National Center for Health Statistics estimates that more than 83,000 deaths per year across all ages and diseases could be prevented if health care disparities were eliminated.[22] Surgical disparities undoubtedly contribute to these national estimates and talks of eliminating health disparities cannot be accomplished without targeted efforts to eliminate disparities in surgery.

Colorectal surgery is where ERAS started and where many surgical disparities exist. Within colorectal surgery, black patients experience worse outcomes in several metrics, including longer length of stay, higher readmission, and higher mortality rates.[14,23–25] In one of the largest studies that included 122,631 patients with colorectal cancer from the Health Cost and Utilization Project Nationwide Inpatient Sample, black patients were more likely to experience in-hospital mortality and longer length of stay when compared with white patients.[26] In another study with 82,474 patients undergoing colorectal surgery, the investigators found that black patients were more likely to undergo open than minimally invasive surgery, with higher mortality and readmission rates compared with similar white patients.[27] The same trends were observed nationally even within surgical diseases like inflammatory bowel disease, with black patients experiencing significantly higher readmission rates (20% vs 15%) and longer lengths of stay (8 vs 6 days) compared with white patients.[25] Studies have shown that these disparities persist despite adjustments for patient-level and procedure-level characteristics, including comorbidities, socioeconomic status, and hospital complexity.[28] Surprisingly, even in the absence of postoperative complications, black race was independently associated with longer postoperative length of stay following colorectal surgery.[29]

Racial/ethnic disparities have also been well described outside of colorectal surgery. Using Medicare data from 1991 to 1994, Lucas and colleagues[30] showed that black patients had an 8% to 57% higher risk for mortality across many surgical specialties/procedures. These included patients undergoing radical cystectomies, pancreatic resections, abdominal aortic aneurysm repairs, coronary artery bypasses, aortic valve replacements, and esophagectomies. In another study conducted on 4725 patients with hepatocellular carcinoma, the investigators found that black patients had higher mortality rates after liver transplantation.[31] In renal transplantation, disparities also exist, with black patients having lower graft survival rates.[32] Black patients are also at increased risk for early death after heart transplantation.[33] Among the pediatric population, black recipients experience less than 50% graft survival for heart transplantation when compared with other racial groups.[34] Overwhelmingly, these studies show that surgical disparities exist and challenge assumptions that we are achieving the best outcome for all patients.

The scope of surgical disparities is large, but frameworks exist to approach it. Studies have shown that health disparities are multifactorial and arise from variations in access and delivery of care at the patient, provider, and health care system level.[21,30,35,36] In collaborations with stakeholders from the NIH and ACS, Haider and colleagues[35] recently identified 5 areas to focus research efforts in surgical disparities: patient factors, provider factors, system and access factors, clinical care and quality factors, and postoperative care and rehabilitation (**Fig. 2**). To eliminate surgical disparities, potential interventions could involve actions such as improving patient-clinician communication with a patient-centered approach, fostering

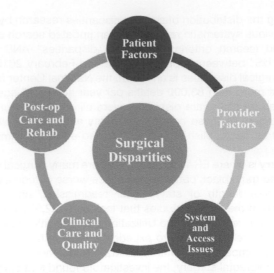

Fig. 2. Thematic framework for conceptualizing surgical disparities. Post-op, postoperative; Rehab, rehabilitation. (*From* Torain MJ, Maragh-Bass AC, Dankwa-Mullen I, et al. surgical disparities: a comprehensive review and new conceptual framework. J Am Coll Surg 2016;223(2):410; with permission.)

engagement and community outreach, improving health care at facilities with higher proportions of minority patients, providing rehabilitation support, and evaluating long-term effects of acute interventions. Ideally, any effective intervention to eliminate surgical disparities would need to be comprehensive in scope and impact patients, providers, and the health care system. Under this framework, ERAS may fulfill many of these requirements.

ENHANCED RECOVERY AFTER SURGERY: A PLATFORM TO ADDRESS DISPARITIES IN SURGERY

ERAS pathways are designed to reduce variations in surgical care through the standardization and implementation of a perioperative care pathway. This design is powerful, effective, and comprehensive. Additionally, ERAS addresses patient-centered issues that patients deem most important in surgical recovery. For example, avoidance of nausea and vomiting are highly desired by patients after major surgery.[37] ERAS offers preventive measures for patients at risk for postoperative nausea and vomiting through preoperative and intraoperative medications, early postoperative ambulation, avoidance of nasogastric tubes, and early advancement of diet. Preoperative counseling and communication, which ERAS emphasizes, is also highly valued by both patients and providers for its role in disseminating information and setting expectations for surgical recovery.[37] Importantly, these patient-centered areas targeted by ERAS overlap with many of the priority areas for interventions described by Haider and colleagues,[35] including patient-clinician communication, engagement, and postoperative support.

Recent studies have begun examining the potential benefits of ERAS in reducing disparities in surgical outcomes among vulnerable populations. Much of the early evidence on ERAS efficacy has been limited to homogeneous patient populations or studies that fail to report racial/ethnic groups. The first study to investigate the potential role of ERAS in reducing racial/ethnic disparities among a large minority population showed that

ERAS eliminated racial/ethnic disparities in postoperative length of stay.[38] In this study, there was a significant disparity in postoperative length of stay among black and white patients before the implementation of ERAS (10.1 vs 7.1 days). After ERAS implementation, black and white patients had similar postoperative length of stay (5.4 vs 5.8 days) without significant increases in postoperative complications or mortality. When adjusting for covariate differences, Wahl and colleagues[38] found that race was no longer associated with prolonged postoperative length of stay in the setting of ERAS. These findings demonstrated the potential efficacy of ERAS in achieving equitable outcomes among a racially diverse surgical population.

Protocol adherence to ERAS components has also been recently studied by race/ ethnicity. In the same study by Wahl and colleagues,[38] black patients were significantly less likely to adhere to preoperative fasting protocols when compared with white patients (32% vs 47%). At another minority-serving institution, Leeds and colleagues[39] also investigated the implementation of ERAS and its effects on minorities. The investigators found no significant difference in complication rates for white and nonwhite surgical patients before and after ERAS and similar overall improvement in the median length of stay for both patient populations. Importantly, racial/ethnic disparities in postoperative length of stay and complication rates were not reported at this single institution even before ERAS implementation, which suggests that equitable surgical care was already present. Before ERAS, for example, the mean length of stay was 5.5 days for white patients and 5.0 days for nonwhites patients; after ERAS implementation both groups had a median length of stay of 4.0 days. This institution's findings are important and demonstrate the benefit of ERAS to all groups. National studies, however, would suggest that major disparities in postoperative length of stay exist in many institutions. Using the American College of Surgeons National Surgical Quality Improvement Program (ACS-NSQIP) database and 140,000 patients undergoing 16 different procedures, Ravi and colleagues[24] found that black patients had significantly higher rates of any postoperative complication (17.0% vs 13.1%) and significantly greater odds of experiencing prolonged length of stay after 10 of the 16 procedures.

Although research to date has often focused on racial/ethnic differences, other types of surgical disparities also exist involving geographic[40] and socioeconomic[36] factors. Geographically, the presence and even use of ERAS varies across health care systems.[41,42] Recent data by the ERAS Compliance Group found that overall ERAS protocol compliance in elective colorectal cancer resections was approximately 75%, but with wide variation between centers and between individual ERAS elements.[43] Studies have shown that patients who live in rural areas experience geographic disparities, including differences in access to care and disease severity at presentation, such as late presentation of colorectal and lung cancers when compared with patients living in urban areas.[40] When considering surgical care for rural populations, the lack of ERAS or poor implementation of ERAS may further drive some of these geographic disparities.

The potential impact of ERAS on surgical disparities is significant. First, ERAS represents a real intervention that is effective in addressing surgical disparities based on published studies. Second, ERAS could serve as a platform or model from which other disparity-reducing interventions could be based. Third, as ERAS diffuses across other institutions and specialties, its impact on vulnerable populations will also continue to grow on a national, and perhaps even global, scale.

Further research is needed to confirm the beneficial effects of ERAS on minority populations and disparities, such as postoperative length of stay. These studies will likely be performed in the next few years, as ERAS-specific data are now being recorded through the ACS-NSQIP.[44] The ERIN initiative (Enhanced Recovery in

NSQIP) is a nationwide unique collaborative of quality improvement that guides the implementation of Enhanced Recovery and audits its implementation by recording specific variables in a robust prospective database.

POTENTIAL MECHANISM(S) BY WHICH ENHANCED RECOVERY AFTER SURGERY MAY REDUCE DISPARITIES

Although the underlying mechanism(s) by which ERAS may reduce disparities is not clear, the standardization of processes and decision-making in surgical care may be an important mechanism. Lau and colleagues[45] demonstrated this concept in addressing the problem of disparities in venous thromboembolism (VTE) prophylaxis. Before any interventions, major disparities in VTE prophylaxis existed with black and white patients receiving standard care 56.6% and 70.1% of the time, respectively, on a trauma service. The same disparity was also present in the medicine service (61.7% vs 69.5%). On mandating and standardizing VTE prophylaxis choices, racial/ethnic disparities were eliminated in both services. This pathway, like ERAS, followed evidence-based algorithms to aid the physician in clinical management. Not surprisingly, when the same care was applied to all patients in the same way, the results were the same across all patients. This finding was replicated in another study that standardized education and phone calls in a health care system to reduce racial/ethnic disparities in hospital utilization among minority groups.[46] In conjunction with the findings on ERAS by Wahl and colleagues,[38] these data suggest that standardization reduces variations in care and has the potential to achieve more equitable care while eliminating previously observed disparities.

Provider bias may be another domain through which ERAS may exert its effects. Provider bias has been shown to play a significant role in determining health outcomes. Specifically, unconscious bias by providers has been associated with negative effects on patient-provider interactions, treatment decisions, and treatment adherence.[47] In surgery, unconscious bias was investigated at Johns Hopkins Hospital using clinical vignettes to survey physicians. The investigators found that race and social biases were present in most responses.[48] By providing a set pathway by which all patients are managed throughout recovery, ERAS may eliminate unconscious, and conscious, biases in management decisions.

FUTURE DIRECTIONS

Surgical care providers need to recognize surgical disparities as a fundamental and preventable problem. A national survey administered to general surgeons found that fewer than one-fourth of surgeons have taken efforts to investigate disparities in their personal practice.[49] Among surgeons who acknowledged it, most believed that racial disparities were due to patient-level factors, including patient attitudes and beliefs (ie, blaming the patient). Despite increasing research on disparities and a call to action by the NIH/ACS, the percentage of surgeons lacking awareness of disparities remains unacceptably high. Providers and the health care system should take responsibility for the elimination of health disparities and the achievement of health equity for our surgical patients. These efforts would additionally support the central aims of the DHHS in their Healthy People 2020 vision to eliminate disparities, address social determinants of health, and improve access to quality health care.[9] As ERAS is increasingly adopted across the world, highlighting its potential role in addressing surgical disparities would be an important way to raise more awareness of this problem.

Understanding the mechanism(s) by which ERAS reduces disparities will enable development of even more effective interventions to improve outcomes. Research in this area should use not only quantitative research, but also consider using qualitative approaches. Qualitative research provides valuable data for designing patient-driven pathways that support differences in needs and expectations toward surgery. These data would also further clarify patient and caregiver factors associated with disparities and be used to inform the development and implementation of more patient-centered interventions.

Future work should also focus on improving ERAS compliance among different populations. Research has shown that overall compliance is associated with improved outcomes following ERAS implementation.[50] When stratified by race/ethnicity, however, Wahl and colleagues[38] showed that overall ERAS adherence varied, with 86.4% adherence in white patients and 76.2% adherence among black patients. In another study, patients with higher socioeconomic status were more likely to be adherent to ERAS protocols.[39] The reason for these disparities in compliance is not yet understood. Lessons learned from studies on compliance with medications in chronic diseases, however, suggest that health literacy (ie, an individual's capacity to obtain, process, and understand health information) may be one potential modifiable reason for poor ERAS compliance.[51] Establishing this relationship(s) among health literacy, ERAS adherence, and surgical outcomes remains largely unexplored.

Technology is another tool that may be leveraged to address surgical disparities. Technology is already in use in for perioperative monitoring and interventions[52] and may prove useful to increase ERAS adherence and potentially improve surgical outcomes. Initial studies using technology in ERAS have been promising. In a study conducted at McGill University, patients undergoing colorectal surgery were instructed to use an application specifically designed to provide daily recovery milestones and achieved 90% compliance with daily questionnaires.[53] At our own institution, recent use of an app-based recovery program has engaged patients, but there appears to be differential initial uptake among different racial/ethnic populations. Although studies have suggested that ERAS compliance varies by race/ethnicity, any efforts to increase compliance across race/ethnic groups could also impact disparities in outcomes. Future studies could leverage the use of technology as strategies to address surgical disparities through increased adherence with ERAS processes.

SUMMARY

Surgical disparities exist. Certain surgical populations suffer from disproportionately worse access, care, and outcomes in surgery. Opportunities exist to better identify, understand, and reduce these disparities. ERAS pathways use standardized perioperative processes and a multidisciplinary philosophy to deliver best-evidence surgical care to *all* patients. As a result, ERAS provides a uniquely pragmatic model for improving outcomes and reducing disparities in disadvantaged surgical populations. In global efforts to achieve health equity, ERAS is one step forward and should become standard of care in surgery.

REFERENCES

1. Gustafsson UO, Scott MJ, Schwenk W, et al. Guidelines for perioperative care in elective colonic surgery: Enhanced Recovery After Surgery (ERAS((R))) Society recommendations. World J Surg 2013;37(2):259–84.
2. Ljungqvist O, Scott M, Fearon KC. Enhanced recovery after surgery: a review. JAMA Surg 2017;152(3):292–8.
3. Grant MC, Yang D, Wu CL, et al. Impact of enhanced recovery after surgery and fast track surgery pathways on healthcare-associated infections: results from a systematic review and meta-analysis. Ann Surg 2017;265(1):68–79.

4. Varadhan KK, Neal KR, Dejong CH, et al. The enhanced recovery after surgery (ERAS) pathway for patients undergoing major elective open colorectal surgery: a meta-analysis of randomized controlled trials. Clin Nutr 2010;29(4):434–40.

5. Kehlet H. Fast-track colorectal surgery. Lancet 2008;371(9615):791–3.

6. Fearon KC, Ljungqvist O, Von Meyenfeldt M, et al. Enhanced recovery after surgery: a consensus review of clinical care for patients undergoing colonic resection. Clin Nutr 2005;24(3):466–77.

7. Lassen K, Soop M, Nygren J, et al. Consensus review of optimal perioperative care in colorectal surgery: Enhanced Recovery After Surgery (ERAS) Group recommendations. Arch Surg 2009;144(10):961–9.

8. Nelson A. Unequal treatment: confronting racial and ethnic disparities in health care. J Natl Med Assoc 2002;94(8):666–8.

9. Services USDoHaH. Healthy people 2020: understanding and improving health. 2nd edition. Washington, DC: U.S. Government Printing Office; 2010.

10. Frieden TR. CDC health disparities and inequalities report - United States, 2013. Foreword. MMWR Suppl 2013;62(3):1–2.

11. Haider AH, Dankwa-Mullan I, Maragh-Bass AC, et al. Setting a national agenda for surgical disparities research: recommendations from the National Institutes of Health and American College of surgeons Summit. JAMA Surg 2016;151(6): 554–63.

12. Meara JG, Leather AJ, Hagander L, et al. Global Surgery 2030: evidence and solutions for achieving health, welfare, and economic development. Int J Obstet Anesth 2016;25:75–8.

13. Healy MA, Mullard AJ, Campbell DA Jr, et al. Hospital and payer costs associated with surgical complications. JAMA Surg 2016;151(9):823–30.

14. Schneider EB, Haider A, Sheer AJ, et al. Differential association of race with treatment and outcomes in Medicare patients undergoing diverticulitis surgery. Arch Surg 2011;146(11):1272–6.

15. Cooper WA, Thourani VH, Guyton RA, et al. Racial disparity persists after on-pump and off-pump coronary artery bypass grafting. Circulation 2009;120(11 Suppl):S59–64.

16. Farjah F, Wood DE, Yanez ND 3rd, et al. Racial disparities among patients with lung cancer who were recommended operative therapy. Arch Surg 2009; 144(1):14–8.

17. Greenstein AJ, Litle VR, Swanson SJ, et al. Racial disparities in esophageal cancer treatment and outcomes. Ann Surg Oncol 2008;15(3):881–8.

18. Pollack CE, Bekelman JE, Epstein AJ, et al. Racial disparities in changing to a high-volume urologist among men with localized prostate cancer. Med Care 2011;49(11):999–1006.

19. Hicks CW, Hashmi ZG, Velopulos C, et al. Association between race and age in survival after trauma. JAMA Surg 2014;149(7):642–7.

20. Singh JA, Lu X, Rosenthal GE, et al. Racial disparities in knee and hip total joint arthroplasty: an 18-year analysis of national Medicare data. Ann Rheum Dis 2014; 73(12):2107–15.

21. Haider AH, Scott VK, Rehman KA, et al. Racial disparities in surgical care and outcomes in the United States: a comprehensive review of patient, provider, and systemic factors. J Am Coll Surg 2013;216(3):482–92.e12.

22. Satcher D, Fryer GE Jr, McCann J, et al. What if we were equal? A comparison of the black-white mortality gap in 1960 and 2000. Health Aff (Millwood) 2005;24(2): 459–64.

23. Schneider EB, Haider AH, Hyder O, et al. Assessing short- and long-term outcomes among black vs white Medicare patients undergoing resection of colorectal cancer. Am J Surg 2013;205(4):402–8.
24. Ravi P, Sood A, Schmid M, et al. Racial/ethnic disparities in perioperative outcomes of major procedures: results from the national surgical quality improvement program. Ann Surg 2015;262(6):955–64.
25. Gunnells DJ Jr, Morris MS, DeRussy A, et al. Racial disparities in readmissions for patients with Inflammatory Bowel Disease (IBD) after colorectal surgery. J Gastrointest Surg 2016;20(5):985–93.
26. Akinyemiju T, Meng Q, Vin-Raviv N. Race/ethnicity and socio-economic differences in colorectal cancer surgery outcomes: analysis of the nationwide inpatient sample. BMC Cancer 2016;16:715.
27. Damle RN, Flahive JM, Davids JS, et al. Examination of racial disparities in the receipt of minimally invasive surgery among a national cohort of adult patients undergoing colorectal surgery. Dis Colon Rectum 2016;59(11):1055–62.
28. Girotti ME, Shih T, Revels S, et al. Racial disparities in readmissions and site of care for major surgery. J Am Coll Surg 2014;218(3):423–30.
29. Giglia MD, DeRussy A, Morris MS, et al. Racial disparities in length-of-stay persist even with no postoperative complications. J Surg Res 2017;214:14–22.
30. Lucas FL, Stukel TA, Morris AM, et al. Race and surgical mortality in the United States. Ann Surg 2006;243(2):281–6.
31. Artinyan A, Mailey B, Sanchez-Luege N, et al. Race, ethnicity, and socioeconomic status influence the survival of patients with hepatocellular carcinoma in the United States. Cancer 2010;116(5):1367–77.
32. Feyssa E, Jones-Burton C, Ellison G, et al. Racial/ethnic disparity in kidney transplantation outcomes: influence of donor and recipient characteristics. J Natl Med Assoc 2009;101(2):111–5.
33. Singh TP, Almond C, Givertz MM, et al. Improved survival in heart transplant recipients in the United States: racial differences in era effect. Circ Heart Fail 2011;4(2):153–60.
34. Mahle WT, Kanter KR, Vincent RN. Disparities in outcome for black patients after pediatric heart transplantation. J Pediatr 2005;147(6):739–43.
35. Torain MJ, Maragh-Bass AC, Dankwa-Mullen I, et al. Surgical disparities: a comprehensive review and new conceptual framework. J Am Coll Surg 2016; 223(2):408–18.
36. Kirby JB, Kaneda T. Unhealthy and uninsured: exploring racial differences in health and health insurance coverage using a life table approach. Demography 2010;47(4):1035–51.
37. Hughes M, Coolsen MM, Aahlin EK, et al. Attitudes of patients and care providers to enhanced recovery after surgery programs after major abdominal surgery. J Surg Res 2015;193(1):102–10.
38. Wahl TS, Goss LE, Morris MS, et al. Enhanced Recovery After Surgery (ERAS) eliminates racial disparities in postoperative length of stay after colorectal surgery. Ann Surg 2017. [Epub ahead of print].
39. Leeds IL, Alimi Y, Hobson DR, et al. Racial and socioeconomic differences manifest in process measure adherence for enhanced recovery after surgery pathway. Dis colon rectum 2017;60(10):1092–101.
40. Paquette I, Finlayson SR. Rural versus urban colorectal and lung cancer patients: differences in stage at presentation. J Am Coll Surg 2007;205(5):636–41.
41. McLeod RS, Aarts MA, Chung F, et al. Development of an enhanced recovery after surgery guideline and implementation strategy based on the knowledge-to-action cycle. Ann Surg 2015;262(6):1016–25.

42. Pedziwiatr M, Kisialeuski M, Wierdak M, et al. Early implementation of Enhanced Recovery After Surgery (ERAS(R)) protocol—compliance improves outcomes: a prospective cohort study. Int J Surg 2015;21:75–81.
43. ERAS Compliance Group. The impact of enhanced recovery protocol compliance on elective colorectal cancer resection: results from an international registry. Ann Surg 2015;261(6):1153–9.
44. Pasquale M, Toselli P, Kolesky R, et al. 2015 Annual NSQIP Presentation presented at ACS (American College of Surgeons) NSQIP (National Surgical Quality Improvement Program) National Conference, ERIN session, Chicago, IL, July 25–28, 2015.
45. Lau BD, Haider AH, Streiff MB, et al. Eliminating healthcare disparities via mandatory clinical decision support: the venous thromboembolism (VTE) example. Med Care 2015;53(1):18–24.
46. Misky GJ, Carlson T, Thompson E, et al. Implementation of an acute venous thromboembolism clinical pathway reduces healthcare utilization and mitigates health disparities. J Hosp Med 2014;9(7):430–5.
47. Hall WJ, Chapman MV, Lee KM, et al. Implicit racial/ethnic bias among health care professionals and its influence on health care outcomes: a systematic review. Am J Public Health 2015;105(12):e60–76.
48. Haider AH, Schneider EB, Sriram N, et al. Unconscious race and social class bias among acute care surgical clinicians and clinical treatment decisions. JAMA Surg 2015;150(5):457–64.
49. Britton BV, Nagarajan N, Zogg CK, et al. Awareness of racial/ethnic disparities in surgical outcomes and care: factors affecting acknowledgment and action. Am J Surg 2016;212(1):102–8.e2.
50. Aarts MA, Rotstein OD, Pearsall EA, et al. Postoperative ERAS interventions have the greatest impact on optimal recovery: experience with implementation of eras across multiple hospitals. Ann Surg 2018;267(6):992–7.
51. Lee YM, Yu HY, You MA, et al. Impact of health literacy on medication adherence in older people with chronic diseases. Collegian 2017;24(1):11–8.
52. Cook DJ, Thompson JE, Prinsen SK, et al. Functional recovery in the elderly after major surgery: assessment of mobility recovery using wireless technology. Ann Thorac Surg 2013;96(3):1057–61.
53. Pecorelli N, Fiore JF Jr, Kaneva P, et al. An app for patient education and self-audit within an enhanced recovery program for bowel surgery: a pilot study assessing validity and usability. Surg Endosc 2017;32(5):2263–73.

Enhanced Recovery After Surgery in Community Hospitals

Amanda Hayman, MD, MPH[a,b,*]

KEYWORDS

- Community hospital • Colon and rectal surgery • Enhanced recovery
- Opiate-sparing

KEY POINTS

- Multidisciplinary collaboration and administrative support are essential to enhanced recovery program (ERP) success.
- The key tenets for ERP are opiate-sparing pain regimen, decreased fasting, and minimizing intravenous fluids.
- Getting buy-in from community surgeons may be difficult due to varied practice patterns and clinical fragmentation.
- Prospective tracking of ERP outcomes will allow for more targeted interventions.

Much of the literature on enhanced recovery programs (ERPs) focuses on implementation at large quaternary academic centers. The most common procedures for ERP implementation, however, are colon and rectal resections. Nationally, more of these procedures are performed in the community, with equivalent survival.[1] Community hospitals face unique challenges, however, that are not always considered in the national discussions surrounding ERP (**Table 1**).

Despite these barriers, many community hospitals have successfully implemented sustainable ERPs within their institutions.[2] There are also strengths to implementing ERPs in a community environment, mostly driven by smaller, more stable, and more intimate clinical teams as well as the greater role that the administration and leadership frequently play as a result of being part of a larger health care system.

Many of the challenges facing community hospitals are shared by those at academic institutions. As a result of financial pressures from declining reimbursements across the health care system, the pressures facing the academic surgeon resemble

Disclosure Statement: The author has nothing to disclose.
a Division of Gastrointestinal and Minimally Invasive Surgery, The Oregon Clinic, 4805 Northeast Glisan Street, Suite 6N60, Portland, OR 97212, USA; b Department of Surgery, Oregon Health & Science University, 3181 SW Sam Jackson Park Road, Portland, OR 97239, USA
* 4805 Northeast Glisan Street, Suite 6N60, Portland, OR 97212.
E-mail address: ahayman@orclinic.com

Surg Clin N Am 98 (2018) 1233–1239
https://doi.org/10.1016/j.suc.2018.07.009
0039-6109/18/© 2018 Elsevier Inc. All rights reserved.

Table 1	
Challenges and strengths of implementing enhanced recovery programs in the community setting	
Challenges	Strengths
• Lack of traditional clinical department structure/leadership • Fragmented care pathways • Low-volume surgeons/hospitals • Surgeons with multiple hospital/health care system affiliations • Financial disincentives to change care pathways • ERP savings directly benefit the hospital system only and not non-hospital employed surgeons • Lack of tangible incentives/enforcement to change physician practice • No/limited trainee coverage	• Less dependence on trainees who have frequent turnover • Smaller institutions with core clinical teams • Health care systems often have multiple hospitals, allowing for a coordinated rollout process system-wide • Administrative champions with interest in quality/process improvement and cost savings • More consistent teams with frequent midlevel providers

those of the community surgeon more than even before. Local health care markets, especially in urban centers, have become increasingly competitive. Many physician reimbursement structures within academic departments have transitioned either partially, via a production bonus, or completely to a relative value unit–based model. These changes, along with increased transparency regarding surgical outcomes and the public availability of clinical data, have forced clinicians to be more responsible for providing efficient and effective care, which is the cornerstone of enhanced recovery. The success of the American College of Surgeons National Surgical Quality Improvement Program (NSQIP) has helped encourage quality improvement efforts worldwide, as has their recently launched Improving Surgical Care and Recovery program that is open to all hospitals nationally, is free of charge, and is aimed at supporting efforts in implementing ERPs (https://qi.facs.org/iscr).

PLANNING AND IMPLEMENTING ENHANCED RECOVERY PROGRAMS IN THE COMMUNITY

The basic actions that are essential to successfully implementing ERPs in the community are outlined.

Step 1: Create a Multidisciplinary Team

Identify physician peer leaders

Forward-thinking health care systems who embark on implementation of an ERP must understand that it requires both an administrative project leader and a dedicated physician champion. There should be a physician champion from each of the relevant disciplines, including surgery and anesthesia, as well as representation from the various nursing phases of care (preoperative, operating room, postanesthesia care unit, and floor), pharmacy, and nutrition. Ideally, the physician leader is currently clinically active and well known and respected in the local surgical community. Clinical demands will be a barrier to multidisciplinary program building, however, and must be anticipated. Therefore, for an ERP rollout to be successful, the health care system should protect time for physician leaders to dedicate themselves to this project. Typically, this is in the form of a medical directorship with an associated stipend or via a consultant role with an hourly stipend. Additionally, aligning the physician leaders with an administrative partner who can serve as a project manager is extremely important for maintaining momentum.

Step 2: Choosing a Bundle: Implications for Community Hospitals

Choosing which elements to include in a specific hospital's bundle depends much on local culture, expertise, and resources. As has been shown previously in surgical site infection reduction, the exact elements of the bundle likely matter less than the process of choosing a bundle that works for an individual center.[3] The 3 common tenets of ERPs are focused on: opiate-sparing pain regimen, decreased fasting, and goal-oriented fluid management (**Fig. 1**).

- Opiate-sparing pain regimen: a common area of debate is which regional anesthesia modality to choose. Options include transversus abduminus plane blocks (with either conventional bupivacaine or liposomal bupivacaine), quadratus lumborum blocks, single-dose intrathecal injection (with morphine or hydromorphone and/or bupivacaine), or epidural catheter-based infusion of opiate and local anesthetic. Although the author's center has had excellent results with intrathecal morphine, implementing this safely requires stringent postprocedure respiratory monitoring to avoid respiratory depression or arrest. This can limit its acceptance at lower volume hospitals with less access to regional anesthesia. Equally important is maximizing the use of narcotic-sparing medications in both the preoperative and postoperative phases of care. These include nonsteroidal anti-inflammatory drugs (NSAIDs) (eg, celecoxib, ketorolac, and ibuprofen), gabapentinoids (gabapentin and pregabalin), and acetaminophen (the author and colleagues recommend oral formulation due to the high cost of intravenous (IV) formulation and its limited clinical benefit over the oral formulation). Sliding scale opiate options then are added, typically tramadol and oxycodone. Any parenteral opiate use, including patient-controlled analgesia, is discouraged and instead initiating oral formulations as soon as possible is recommended.
- Decreased fasting time: American Society of Anesthesiologists guidelines allow elective, healthy patients to take in clear liquids up to 2 hours prior to surgery.[4] The author and colleagues have changed this to 4 hours prior, to allow for surgery

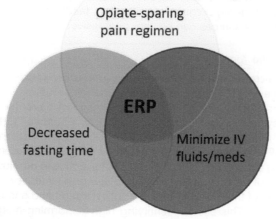

Fig. 1. Core principles of ERPs.

scheduling move ups. Postoperatively, the author's patients start clear liquids the night of surgery. The nursing-led protocol allows patients to advance to a fiber-restricted diet either postoperative day 0 or day 1. Immunonutrition drinks (protein drinks containing arginine) also are provided for all major abdominal surgical patients at nutritional risk in both the preoperative and postoperative time periods. The author and colleagues have had strong input from the nutrition department about this process.

- Goal-oriented fluid management: although many studies discuss goal-directed approaches, in all practicality, finding the true fluid state of a patient can be challenging. Most elective colorectal resections can be approached via minimally invasive techniques with minimal blood loss with few perioperative fluid shifts, despite preoperative mechanical bowel preparation. It is also important for anesthetists to keep in mind that, despite the presence of a urinary catheter, most colon and rectal resections are performed in lithotomy and steep Trendelenburg position with the catheter over the leg, which can lead to falsely low urine output readings. Therefore, the author and colleagues set a goal crystalloid fluid replacement of approximately 500 mL per hour for routine cases. Postoperatively, the author and colleagues give 40 mL of crystalloid per hour until the next morning when all IV fluids are then stopped.

Step 3: Getting Buy-in from the Nonemployed Physician

Because many private practitioners still function in a fee-for-service model, their presence at monthly departmental meetings or morbidity and mortality conferences may be limited because they may be seen as not revenue generating. Therefore, it can be difficult to disseminate changes in care processes in such a fragmented system.

The author and colleagues have found the most effective method of promoting change is to engage individual providers on their own turf, that is, via peer-to-peer discussions at their clinic or during administrative or business meetings. These smaller venues promote more nuanced discussions that can better identify provider concerns and thus barriers to implementation. However, person meetings can be time intensive on the part of the providers but will likely be the most effective way to induce change. Also, surgeons respond to data. If there are provider concerns about specific elements of the enhanced recovery bundle, the physician leader should provide studies that refute their colleagues' concerns. It is essential to provide data on surgical outcomes to the local providers after implementation in order to demonstrate that ERPs are safe and effective. Lastly, giving surgeon-specific data feedback to providers based on NSQIP or internal data sources can be very persuasive.

Step 4: Providing the Tools for Success

Harnessing the electronic medical records: physician order sets

To ensure a successful ERP, the care bundle changes must be ingrained in a physician's daily work flow. Community surgeons may not have the same electronic medical record system in their outpatient setting as a hospital, further fragmenting patient care and making it more difficult to track ERP metric compliance. Because many of the ERP measures are implemented during the inpatient hospital stay, however, creating evidenced-based order sets for both the preoperative and postoperative phases of care is essential. In the author's institution, it is possible to track the utilization of the ERP order set by both surgeon and hospital over the system's 53 institutions. This allows identifying high-performing hospitals as well as those hospitals that could benefit from further education.

Providing patient resources to physicians

Although setting patient expectations about the ERP hospital experience and discharge planning is essential to success, the additional time and resources it takes to prepare a patient is a major barrier to surgeon buy-in. Therefore, it behooves a hospital system to provide multimedia patient resources to support surgeons' efforts. If a center has a robust preoperative clinic, this is an ideal environment to provide these materials. The author and colleagues have created colorectal ERP-specific patient folders that contain preoperative, in-hospital, and postdischarge instructions and guidelines and also created an online video that reviews similar information and which can be found on the hospital system Web site.

Step 5: Sustaining Success

Track clinical outcomes over time

After implementation, the project manager should provide ongoing feedback to the hospitals on their performance. Because surgeons by nature are competitive, comparing individual surgeon outcomes and compliance with ERP measures with their own historical outcomes or with their peers can be a strong motivating factor. Furthermore, providing evidence that ERP implementation will not adversely affect their patients' outcomes is equally important. Therefore, regular feedback to providers and care teams about their performance will help ensure ongoing compliance with the program (**Table 2**).

Care team reminders

Given the reality of frequent bedside provider turnover, after the initial rollout, it is important for ERP leaders to circle back to the clinical teams on at least an annual basis with updates, reminders, and patient outcomes to support ongoing ERP compliance. This can be done via continuing education unit seminars, grand rounds, or smaller, more informal information sessions on the wards.

Predicting barriers and risks of failure

Understanding the local culture as well as resource and logistical limitations is essential to creating a realistic and practical ERP for each center. Some customization for a system's ERP may be necessary. Examples of barriers the author and colleagues encountered when rolling out an ERP are limited nursing staffing for high-acuity postoperative patient needs on the surgical ward at smaller hospitals (ie, insulin drips or continuous pulse oximetry for respiratory depression after intrathecal administration), getting immunonutrition drinks on the inpatient and outpatient formulary, pharmacy budget restraints around proprietary medications (eg, liposomal bupivacaine, parenteral acetaminophen/ibuprofen, and alvimopan), expertise and acceptance of regional anesthesia, and absence of an established and comprehensive preoperative clinic.

Lastly, knowing when a patient is not a good ERP candidate is essential. Especially early on during implementation, if a patient experiences a complication that could be related to ERP (renal insufficiency or bleeding from NSAIDs, respiratory depression from intrathecal analgesia, aspiration from early feeding in presence of an ileus, or early postoperative readmission), this can threaten ERP acceptance among the clinical team. Examples of patients who are likely poor ERP candidates include nonelective patients (ie, acute bowel obstruction or emergent procedure) and elderly, disabled, altered mental status, or renal failure patients.

It is important, however, to reiterate to the surgical community that although many of the patients may not be good candidates for all the ERP components, it is likely that some of the core ERP principles can safely be applied to most patients. As knowledge and acceptance of ERP spreads, the steps described hopefully can guide community

Table 2
Regional surgical outcomes over time after ERP implementation

N	2014			2015			2016			2017		
	A	B	C	A	B	C	A	B	C	A	B	C
Volume	272	219	22	253	180	18	239	191	20	237	200	17
Length of stay (days)	5	4	6	4	4	6	4	3	5	4	3	4
30-day readmissions, N (%)	29 (11%)	0 (0%)	0 (0%)	24 (9%)	3 (17%)	3 (17%)	30 (13%)	1 (5%)	4 (20%)	18 (9%)	3 (18%)	3 (18%)
30-day reoperations, N (%)	15 (6%)	9 (4%)	0 (0%)	10 (4%)	6 (3%)	0 (0%)	14 (6%)	3 (2%)	2 (10%)	5 (2%)	4 (2%)	1 (6%)

Abbreviations: A/B, high-volume urban hospital; C, low-volume suburban hospital.

hospitals in their efforts to implement ERP and help improve patient outcomes and preoperative experiences, while concomitantly providing cost savings as a result of reduced resource utilization and decreased hospital length of stay.

REFERENCES

1. Veenstra CM, Epstein AJ, Liao K, et al. Hospital academic status and value of care for nometastatic colon cancer. J Oncol Pract 2015;11(3):e304–12.
2. Geltzeiler CB, Rotramel A, Wilson C, et al. Prospective study of colorectal enhanced recovery after surgery in a community hospital. JAMA Surg 2014; 149(9):955–61.
3. Tanner J, Padley W, Assadian O, et al. Do surgical care bundle reduce the risk of surgical site infections in patients undergoing colorectal surgery? A systematic review and cohort meta-analysis of 8,515 patients. Surgery 2015;138(1):66–77.
4. American Society of Anesthesiologists Committee. Practice guidelines for preoperative fasting and the use of pharmacologic agents to reduce the risk of pulmonary aspiration: application to healthy patients undergoing elective procedures: an updated report by the American Society of Anesthesiologists Committee on standards and practice parameters. Anesthesiology 2011;3(114):495–511.

Enhanced Recovery After Surgery
Recent Developments in Colorectal Surgery

Jim P. Tiernan, MD, PhD, FRCS, David Liska, MD*

KEYWORDS

- Enhanced recovery • Fast-track surgery • Colorectal • Innovation

KEY POINTS

- Enhanced recovery after surgery (ERAS) has been established as a safe and effective tool for early recovery and discharge after colorectal resection.
- ERAS protocol compliance seems to be an essential factor associated with optimal recovery.
- Personalized analgesia via pharmacogenetic testing may be a promising addition to ERAS protocols.
- The value of gum chewing, carbohydrate loading, immunonutrition, and routine application of epidural analgesia and goal-directed fluid therapy have all been questioned in recent publications, necessitating further studies to guide personalized, value-based interventions.

INTRODUCTION

The benefits of careful analgesia management, early oral feeding, and early mobilization after colorectal resection were first described more than 20 years ago.[1–3] When combined with laparoscopic resection, length of hospital stay was reduced to just 2 days,[4] a huge paradigm shift from traditional open resection and delayed oral feeding, where typical length of stay was up to 12 days.[5] Since then, the concept of fast-track surgery, or enhanced recovery after surgery (ERAS), has been adopted by the global colorectal surgical community, with the support of anesthesiologists, operating room teams, nurses, and allied health care professionals. Initial concerns around secondary increases in complication rates were not borne out: a meta-analysis of randomized trials confirmed that ERAS reduced overall morbidity and length of stay without increasing readmission rates.[6] ERAS has also complemented

Disclosure statement: The authors have nothing to disclose.
Department of Colorectal Surgery, Digestive Disease and Surgery Institute, Cleveland Clinic, 9500 Euclid Avenue, A30, Cleveland, OH 44195, USA
* Corresponding author.
E-mail address: liskad@ccf.org

Surg Clin N Am 98 (2018) 1241–1249
https://doi.org/10.1016/j.suc.2018.07.010
0039-6109/18/© 2018 Elsevier Inc. All rights reserved.

the uptake of minimally invasive resection, where randomized studies have shown gains in terms of hospital stay, and immune response are greater than with open resection.[7,8] A challenge for researchers has been to establish the relative effects of the individual components of ERAS protocols, an inherent problem with a multimodal intervention. This article reviews some of the newer interventions, controversies, and latest refinements to ERAS protocols in colorectal surgery.

METHODS

A detailed search of PubMed, Embase and Cochrane databases was undertaken by 2 independent reviewers to identify relevant literature in English relating to ERAS and colorectal surgery. The initial keywords used were "enhanced recovery" AND/OR "fast-track surgery" AND "abdominal" OR "colorectal" OR "gastrointestinal." Further searches were performed by cross-referencing articles.

RESULTS
Preoperative

Carbohydrate loading
Insulin resistance is known to adversely affect morbidity and mortality in critically unwell patients and has been shown to independently predict length of stay in surgical patients. Ljungqvist and colleagues[9] postulated that preventing or treating insulin resistance associated with surgical stress would influence the surgical outcome, leading to the avoidance of fasting and preoperative carbohydrate loading being incorporated into ERAS care bundles.[10,11] Several randomized trials attempted to assess the individual benefit of carbohydrate loading and a Cochrane review in 2014[12] found that although there was no differences in complication rates associated with carbohydrate loading, there was a small decrease in length of stay. This could be attributed, however, to a lack of appropriate blinding, leading to potential bias. A recent network meta-analysis included 43 trials involving more than 3110 patients compared both low-dose and high-dose carbohydrate loading with water and placebo in an elegantly designed multiple-treatment analysis. There was no statistically significant difference in the rates of postoperative complications or in most of the secondary outcomes between treatment and control groups; there was a small advantage in length of hospital stay compared with fasting but not compared with water or placebo.[13] There are few data on the safety and efficacy of carbohydrate loading in patients with diabetes.[14]

Immunonutrition
Another preoperative nutritional intervention that has gained attention in those designing ERAS pathways is the concept of immunonutrition. Immune-modulating substrates, such as arginine, glutamine, and omega-3 fatty acids, have been linked in early studies to decreased infective complications, shorter length of stay, and preservation of small bowel function.[15] Subsequent studies have shown overall benefit: a randomized controlled trial by Moya and colleagues[16] included 128 patients and showed a decrease in wound infection rate with immunonutrition. A population database analysis of 772 patients showed there were significantly fewer readmissions and a decreased risk of both wound infection and thromboembolism with arginine-based immunonutrition.[17] This translated into substantial cost savings. A prospective cohort study of 3375 patients from Washington State did not show a significant difference in the rate of serious adverse events, but after propensity matching, the rate of prolonged length of stay (defined as >1.5-times the median length of stay) was significantly lower

in those receiving 5 days of preoperative immunonutrition.[18] An acknowledged limitation of this study and other studies on immunonutrition is the lack of a reliable measure of patient compliance, introducing the potential for bias.

Bowel preparation

Although many enhanced recovery pathways (ERPs) call for the omission of routine bowel preparation, more recently the majority opinion in the United States has returned to recommending the routine use of a combined mechanical bowel preparation (MBP) with oral antibiotics before elective colorectal surgery. Due to conflicting studies—with small but important differences in design—this is still a matter of controversy with divergent practices and opinions between the United States and Europe. Observational studies in the United States have suggested advantages in combining MBP with oral antibiotics that include lower rates of surgical site infections, shorter postoperative length of stay, and reduced readmission rates.[19,20] Kiran and coworkers[21] showed, in a National Surgical Quality Improvement Program study examining more than 8000 patients, that the group who had both MBP with oral antibiotics had an approximately 50% reduction in surgical site infections, anastomotic leak, and ileus.

Epidural and regional analgesia

Perioperative multimodal analgesia is an important component of ERPs. The goal of multimodal analgesia is to achieve pain relief with minimal opiate consumption, using combinations of analgesic medications that act on different sites and pathways in an additive or synergistic manner. Local anesthetic infusion via thoracic epidural anesthesia has long been recommended as the gold standard in open colorectal surgery, with numerous studies showing benefits over intravenous opioid analgesia.[22,23] These benefits have not been observed, however, after laparoscopic surgery, particularly for patients treated within the context of an enhanced recovery pathway.[24,25] Furthermore, hypotension, urinary retention, and pruritus are common side effects associated with thoracic epidural anesthesia. For these reasons, recent attention has shifted to the use of transversus abdominis plane (TAP) blocks as a valuable component of multimodal analgesia. The TAP block was first described in 2001 by Rafi[26] and infiltrates local anesthetic into the neurovascular plane between the internal oblique and transversus abdominis muscle. Several studies and meta-analyses indicate that TAP blocks or TAP catheters for abdominal surgical procedures are associated with superior analgesia and decreased postoperative opioid consumption compared with opioid analgesia alone.[27,28] In a small randomized double-blind prospective trial, Keller and colleagues[29] demonstrated that TAP blocks improve immediate short-term opioid use and pain outcomes but do not lead to lower overall opioid use, shorter hospital stay, and lower readmission rate. A recently published meta-analysis on the efficacy of TAP blocks using short-acting local anesthetics in laparoscopic colorectal surgery, including 452 patients from 6 studies, found that the TAP block had a significant effect on the postoperative pain outcome in the early (0-h to 2-h) and late (24-h) period at movement. It did not, however, have a significant effect on the postoperative opioid consumption or pain outcome in the early and late periods at rest.[30] Liposomal bupivacaine for TAP blocks shows some promise for longer-term postoperative analgesia[31] via a delayed release mechanism; however, there are no large-scale randomized controlled trials to guide practice or to definitively demonstrate the analgesic efficacy and value of this intervention.

Intraoperative

Goal-directed fluid management

The impact of changes in intraoperative volume status on gastrointestinal mucosa has been suggested as a cause of delayed return of bowel function postoperatively,[32] leading to the concept of goal-directed fluid therapy (GDFT). Traditionally, intraoperative oliguria was seen as a proxy for hypovolemia and renal hypoperfusion, triggering augmentation of intravenous fluid therapy. It is now understood, however, that oliguria can be a normal physiologic response to anesthesia and surgery and, therefore, should not be used, in isolation, as assessment of volume status.[33] Measurements of stroke volume and cardiac output using various minimally invasive techniques have been used to guide intraoperative fluid requirements.[34] Initial trials were promising, suggesting a shorter length of stay and a reduction on postoperative complications.[35,36] A recent meta-analysis, including 23 studies and 2099 patients, found that GDFT was associated with a significant reduction in morbidity, length of stay, and time to bowel movement but no difference in mortality or risk of paralytic ileus.[37] There was a difference on subgroup analysis between those patients managed in an ERAS pathway and those not: for ERAS patients, the only benefits were reduction in length of intensive treatment unit stay and time to first bowel movement (but not ileus), whereas for those not managed as part of an ERAS pathway, there were significant advantages in overall morbidity and overall length of stay. The investigators concluded that GDFT might not benefit all patients undergoing elective surgery, in particular those enrolled in an ERAS pathway. This raises the question of cost-effectiveness when routinely incorporating GDFT into such pathways. In a new development in this field, Asklid and colleagues[38] have shown a possible association between restrictive perioperative fluid therapy and 5-year survival in a Swedish database analysis of 911 patients. Although the mechanistic basis is unclear, further evaluation is required.

Dedicated operating room teams

Investigators have sought to study the variability in outcomes and discrepancy in treatment effects after ERAS protocols. A novel strand of investigation has been the perioperative team. Grant and colleagues[39] hypothesized that intraoperative provider team networks, consisting of surgeons, anesthesiologists, and certified registered nurse anesthetists, would affect network centrality (the importance of a team member in the network) and, therefore, clinical outcomes. They concluded that dedicated teams improved centrality, leading to significantly improved clinical outcomes, including ERAS compliance, length of stay, surgical site infection, and risk of return to the operating room.

Training and implementation

Another line of investigation to reduce variability in ERAS protocols has been training. Recent work on this topic has involved the development of a consensus on the training required. A group of European collaborators, all experts in ERAS provision, used a modified Delphi methodology to develop an ERAS training curriculum, a framework for successful implementation and methods for assessing effectiveness.[40] This has the potential to make ERAS adoption more accessible and provide a degree of standardization to provision.

Postoperative

Chewing gum

Several trials suggested chewing gum postoperatively led to earlier return of bowel function and a reduced length of stay. A Cochrane review confirmed small benefits on meta-analysis but the quality of the trials was poor with generally small sample sizes.[41] A large, high-quality, multicenter randomized controlled trial has recently been published by de Leede and colleagues[42] evaluating gum chewing in the setting of ERAS-based postoperative care. The trial was powered to detect a difference in length of stay of 1 day, leading to an impressive 1000 patients in each study arm. The investigators found no significant difference in length of stay, time to flatus, time to defecation, or rate of complications up to 30 days.

Personalized analgesia

The field of pharmacogenetics is relatively new and timely given the overuse of narcotics in secondary care, contributing to the current opioid epidemic. It also sits well with the ongoing drive for personalized therapeutics in all fields of medicine. It relies on the premise that mutations in certain genes result in a variable response to analgesics at the individual patient level,[43] in particular nonsteroidal anti-inflammatories and opiate analgesics. Senagore and colleagues[44] evaluated 63 consecutive patients undergoing elective colorectal or ventral hernia surgery and compared them to a historical control group undergoing the same operations as part of an ERAS pathway. The study group underwent genetic testing for CYP1A2, CYP2C19, CYP2C9, CYP2D6, CYP3A4, CYP3A5, COMT, OPRM1, and ABCB1 genes and the results were used to produce individualized analgesia regimens. The investigators reported a 50% reduction in narcotic consumption compared with the control group and fewer analgesic-related side effects. Although the study is limited by a small sample size and a nonrandomized design, the results are promising from surgical, economic, and public health perspectives.

Early discharge: how early is safe?

As ERAS protocols have become the standard of care, efforts have been made to explore the limits of safe discharge. Keller and colleagues[45,46] identified length of operation, presence of comorbidities, and a modified frailty index of 2 as risk factors for failing early discharge, defined as within 3 days of operation. Lawrence and colleagues[47] conducted a retrospective review of all major resections performed by a single surgeon over a 5-year period and found that those discharged between 24 hours and 48 hours postoperatively (234 patients) were not at an increased risk for readmission. Managing patient expectations by identifying those at risk of failing early discharge may be key to avoiding failure or readmission.

Some investigators have advocated the use of inflammatory markers, such as procalcitonin or C-reactive protein (CRP), as markers of safe discharge.[48,49] CRP was reported to have a negative predictive value of 96.9% (cutoff <2.7 ng/mL) on postoperative day 3 and 98.3% (cutoff 2.3 ng/mL) on postoperative day 5 for excluding an anastomotic leak. Calcitonin performed similarly. CRP is widely available and relatively cheap and could add to the clinical assessment and subsequent decision making regarding when is safe to discharge.

μ-Opioid receptor antagonists

Alvimopan and methylnaltrexone are both peripheral μ-antagonists that are Food and Drug Administration approved for the treatment of gastrointestinal dysfunction: alvimopan for postoperative ileus and methylnaltrexone for opioid-induced constipation. Several randomized trials have evaluated alvimopan in major open abdominal and colorectal surgery,[50–52] with the vast majority showing clinical benefit in terms of incidence of both upper and lower gastrointestinal symptoms of ileus and significant reduction in length of stay of almost 1 day. Cost-effectiveness has been a persistent concern, although a recent cost-effectiveness model analysis suggested overall benefit.[53] Further studies are needed on the benefits and value of μ-opioid receptor antagonists in patients undergoing laparoscopic surgery or colorectal resections with a diverting ostomy.

Impact of Individual Enhanced Recovery After Surgery Interventions

Several recent articles have attempted to quantify the impact of individual components of ERAS bundles on clinical outcomes. Jurt and colleagues[54] retrospectively assessed more than 300 colorectal patients treated consecutively using an ERAS approach and concluded that minimally invasive surgery is the single most important factor. Greater adherence to the protocol was associated with improved outcomes. Pisarska and colleagues[55] conducted a similar study but divided patients into 3 groups according to how compliant their care had been with the 16 components of their ERAS protocol. They found that full compliance with the protocol was associated with better outcomes even when compared with those who were compliant with 70% to 90% of the bundle. A systematic review of factors predicting outcome in laparoscopic colorectal ERAS surgery confirmed compliance as the most frequently reported predictive factor.[56] Most recently Aarts and colleagues[57] analyzed 2876 colorectal patients enrolled in ERAS programs across 15 hospitals. They found compliance most strongly associated with optimal recovery and that the biggest impact was seen in patients operated via the open approach.

SUMMARY

ERAS has been established as a safe and effective tool in optimizing recovery. The evidence base for individual components of bundles is increasing in volume and quality, leading to exciting avenues of new research and the removal of interventions without benefit.

REFERENCES

1. Bradshaw BG, Liu SS, Thirlby RC. Standardized perioperative care protocols and reduced length of stay after colon surgery. J Am Coll Surg 1998;186(5):501–6.
2. Liu SS, Carpenter RL, Mackey DC, et al. Effects of perioperative analgesic technique on rate of recovery after colon surgery. Anesthesiology 1995;83(4):757–65.
3. Moiniche S, Bulow S, Hesselfeldt P, et al. Convalescence and hospital stay after colonic surgery with balanced analgesia, early oral feeding, and enforced mobilisation. Eur J Surg 1995;161(4):283–8.
4. Bardram L, Funch-Jensen P, Jensen P, et al. Recovery after laparoscopic colonic surgery with epidural analgesia, and early oral nutrition and mobilisation. Lancet 1995;345(8952):763–4.
5. Bokey EL, Chapuis PH, Fung C, et al. Postoperative morbidity and mortality following resection of the colon and rectum for cancer. Dis Colon Rectum 1995; 38(5):480–6 [discussion: 6–7].
6. Greco M, Capretti G, Beretta L, et al. Enhanced recovery program in colorectal surgery: a meta-analysis of randomized controlled trials. World J Surg 2014; 38(6):1531–41.
7. Veenhof AA, Vlug MS, van der Pas MH, et al. Surgical stress response and postoperative immune function after laparoscopy or open surgery with fast track or standard perioperative care: a randomized trial. Ann Surg 2012;255(2):216–21.
8. Vlug MS, Wind J, Hollmann MW, et al. Laparoscopy in combination with fast track multimodal management is the best perioperative strategy in patients undergoing colonic surgery: a randomized clinical trial (LAFA-study). Ann Surg 2011;254(6): 868–75.
9. Ljungqvist O, Nygren J, Thorell A. Modulation of post-operative insulin resistance by pre-operative carbohydrate loading. Proc Nutr Soc 2002;61(3):329–36.

10. Ljungqvist O. Modulating postoperative insulin resistance by preoperative carbohydrate loading. Best Pract Res Clin Anaesthesiol 2009;23(4):401–9.
11. Nygren J. The metabolic effects of fasting and surgery. Best Pract Res Clin anaesthesiology 2006;20(3):429–38.
12. Smith MD, McCall J, Plank L, et al. Preoperative carbohydrate treatment for enhancing recovery after elective surgery. Cochrane Database Syst Rev 2014;(8):CD009161.
13. Amer MA, Smith MD, Herbison GP, et al. Network meta-analysis of the effect of preoperative carbohydrate loading on recovery after elective surgery. Br J Surg 2017;104(3):187–97.
14. Gustafsson UO, Nygren J, Thorell A, et al. Pre-operative carbohydrate loading may be used in type 2 diabetes patients. Acta Anaesthesiol Scand 2008;52(7): 946–51.
15. Zheng YM, Li F, Zhang MM, et al. Glutamine dipeptide for parenteral nutrition in abdominal surgery: a meta-analysis of randomized controlled trials. World J Gastroenterol 2006;12(46):7537–41.
16. Moya P, Miranda E, Soriano-Irigaray L, et al. Perioperative immunonutrition in normo-nourished patients undergoing laparoscopic colorectal resection. Surg Endosc 2016;30(11):4946–53.
17. Banerjee S, Garrison LP, Danel A, et al. Effects of arginine-based immunonutrition on inpatient total costs and hospitalization outcomes for patients undergoing colorectal surgery. Nutrition 2017;42:106–13.
18. Thornblade LW, Varghese TK Jr, Shi X, et al. Preoperative immunonutrition and elective colorectal resection outcomes. Dis Colon Rectum 2017;60(1):68–75.
19. Cannon JA, Altom LK, Deierhoi RJ, et al. Preoperative oral antibiotics reduce surgical site infection following elective colorectal resections. Dis Colon Rectum 2012;55(11):1160–6.
20. Toneva GD, Deierhoi RJ, Morris M, et al. Oral antibiotic bowel preparation reduces length of stay and readmissions after colorectal surgery. J Am Coll Surg 2013;216(4):756–62 [discussion: 62–3].
21. Kiran RP, Murray AC, Chiuzan C, et al. Combined preoperative mechanical bowel preparation with oral antibiotics significantly reduces surgical site infection, anastomotic leak, and ileus after colorectal surgery. Ann Surg 2015;262(3):416–25 [discussion: 23–5].
22. Pöpping DM, Elia N, Van Aken HK, et al. Impact of epidural analgesia on mortality and morbidity after surgery: systematic review and meta-analysis of randomized controlled trials. Ann Surg 2014;259(6):1056–67.
23. Feldheiser A, Aziz O, Baldini G, et al. Enhanced Recovery After Surgery (ERAS) for gastrointestinal surgery, part 2: consensus statement for anaesthesia practice. Acta Anaesthesiol Scand 2016;60(3):289–334.
24. Levy BF, Scott MJ, Fawcett W, et al. Randomized clinical trial of epidural, spinal or patient-controlled analgesia for patients undergoing laparoscopic colorectal surgery. Br J Surg 2011;98(8):1068–78.
25. Hübner M, Blanc C, Roulin D, et al. Randomized clinical trial on epidural versus patient-controlled analgesia for laparoscopic colorectal surgery within an enhanced recovery pathway. Ann Surg 2015;261(4):648–53.
26. Rafi AN. Abdominal field block: a new approach via the lumbar triangle. Anaesthesia 2001;56(10):1024–6.
27. Baeriswyl M, Kirkham KR, Kern C, et al. The analgesic efficacy of ultrasound-guided transversus abdominis plane block in adult patients: a meta-analysis. Anesth Analg 2015;121(6):1640–54.

28. Zhao X, Tong Y, Ren H, et al. Transversus abdominis plane block for postoperative analgesia after laparoscopic surgery: a systematic review and meta-analysis. Int J Clin Exp Med 2014;7(9):2966–75.

29. Keller DS, Ermlich BO, Schiltz N, et al. The effect of transversus abdominis plane blocks on postoperative pain in laparoscopic colorectal surgery: a prospective, randomized, double-blind trial. Dis Colon Rectum 2014;57(11):1290–7.

30. Oh TK, Lee SJ, Do SH, et al. Transversus abdominis plane block using a short-acting local anesthetic for postoperative pain after laparoscopic colorectal surgery: a systematic review and meta-analysis. Surg Endosc 2018; 32(2):545–52.

31. Stokes AL, Adhikary SD, Quintili A, et al. Liposomal bupivacaine use in transversus abdominis plane blocks reduces pain and postoperative intravenous opioid requirement after colorectal surgery. Dis Colon Rectum 2017;60(2):170–7.

32. Holland J, Carey M, Hughes N, et al. Intraoperative splanchnic hypoperfusion, increased intestinal permeability, down-regulation of monocyte class II major histocompatibility complex expression, exaggerated acute phase response, and sepsis. Am J Surg 2005;190(3):393–400.

33. Egal M, de Geus HR, van Bommel J, et al. Targeting oliguria reversal in perioperative restrictive fluid management does not influence the occurrence of renal dysfunction: A systematic review and meta-analysis. Eur J Anaesthesiol 2016; 33(6):425–35.

34. Funk DJ, Moretti EW, Gan TJ. Minimally invasive cardiac output monitoring in the perioperative setting. Anesth Analg 2009;108(3):887–97.

35. Abbas SM, Hill AG. Systematic review of the literature for the use of oesophageal Doppler monitor for fluid replacement in major abdominal surgery. Anaesthesia 2008;63(1):44–51.

36. Harten J, Crozier JE, McCreath B, et al. Effect of intraoperative fluid optimisation on renal function in patients undergoing emergency abdominal surgery: a randomised controlled pilot study (ISRCTN 11799696). Int J Surg 2008;6(3): 197–204.

37. Rollins KE, Lobo DN. Intraoperative goal-directed fluid therapy in elective major abdominal surgery: a meta-analysis of randomized controlled trials. Ann Surg 2016;263(3):465–76.

38. Asklid D, Segelman J, Gedda C, et al. The impact of perioperative fluid therapy on short-term outcomes and 5-year survival among patients undergoing colorectal cancer surgery - a prospective cohort study within an ERAS protocol. Eur J Surg Oncol 2017;43(8):1433–9.

39. Grant MC, Hanna A, Benson A, et al. Dedicated operating room teams and clinical outcomes in an enhanced recovery after surgery pathway for colorectal surgery. J Am Coll Surg 2018;226(3):267–76.

40. Francis NK, Walker T, Carter F, et al. Consensus on training and implementation of enhanced recovery after surgery: a delphi study. World J Surg 2018;42(7): 1919–28.

41. Pereira Gomes Morais E, Riera R, Porfirio GJ, et al. Chewing gum for enhancing early recovery of bowel function after caesarean section. Cochrane Database Syst Rev 2016;(10):CD011562.

42. de Leede EM, van Leersum NJ, Kroon HM, et al. Multicentre randomized clinical trial of the effect of chewing gum after abdominal surgery. Br J Surg 2018;105(7): 820–8.

43. Ko TM, Wong CS, Wu JY, et al. Pharmacogenomics for personalized pain medicine. Acta Anaesthesiol Taiwan 2016;54(1):24–30.

44. Senagore AJ, Champagne BJ, Dosokey E, et al. Pharmacogenetics-guided analgesics in major abdominal surgery: further benefits within an enhanced recovery protocol. Am J Surg 2017;213(3):467–72.
45. Keller DS, Bankwitz B, Woconish D, et al. Predicting who will fail early discharge after laparoscopic colorectal surgery with an established enhanced recovery pathway. Surg Endosc 2014;28(1):74–9.
46. Keller DS, Bankwitz B, Nobel T, et al. Using frailty to predict who will fail early discharge after laparoscopic colorectal surgery with an established recovery pathway. Dis Colon Rectum 2014;57(3):337–42.
47. Lawrence JK, Keller DS, Samia H, et al. Discharge within 24 to 72 hours of colorectal surgery is associated with low readmission rates when using enhanced recovery pathways. J Am Coll Surg 2013;216(3):390–4.
48. Giaccaglia V, Salvi PF, Antonelli MS, et al. Procalcitonin reveals early dehiscence in colorectal surgery: the PREDICS study. Ann Surg 2016;263(5):967–72.
49. Dupre A, Gagniere J, Samba H, et al. CRP predicts safe patient discharge after colorectal surgery. Ann Surg 2018;267(2):e33.
50. Ludwig K, Enker WE, Delaney CP, et al. Gastrointestinal tract recovery in patients undergoing bowel resection: results of a randomized trial of alvimopan and placebo with a standardized accelerated postoperative care pathway. Arch Surg 2008;143(11):1098–105.
51. Viscusi ER, Goldstein S, Witkowski T, et al. Alvimopan, a peripherally acting mu-opioid receptor antagonist, compared with placebo in postoperative ileus after major abdominal surgery: results of a randomized, double-blind, controlled study. Surg Endosc 2006;20(1):64–70.
52. Delaney CP, Weese JL, Hyman NH, et al. Phase III trial of alvimopan, a novel, peripherally acting, mu opioid antagonist, for postoperative ileus after major abdominal surgery. Dis Colon Rectum 2005;48(6):1114–25 [discussion: 25–6]; [author reply: 27–9].
53. Earnshaw SR, Kauf TL, McDade C, et al. Economic impact of alvimopan considering varying definitions of postoperative ileus. J Am Coll Surg 2015;221(5):941–50.
54. Jurt J, Slieker J, Frauche P, et al. Enhanced recovery after surgery: can we rely on the key factors or do we need the bel ensemble? World J Surg 2017;41(10):2464–70.
55. Pisarska M, Pedziwiatr M, Malczak P, et al. Do we really need the full compliance with ERAS protocol in laparoscopic colorectal surgery? A prospective cohort study. Int J Surg 2016;36(Pt A):377–82.
56. Messenger DE, Curtis NJ, Jones A, et al. Factors predicting outcome from enhanced recovery programmes in laparoscopic colorectal surgery: a systematic review. Surg Endosc 2017;31(5):2050–71.
57. Aarts MA, Rotstein OD, Pearsall EA, et al. Postoperative ERAS interventions have the greatest impact on optimal recovery: experience with implementation of ERAS across multiple hospitals. Ann Surg 2018;267(6):992–7.

Enhanced Recovery After Surgery: Hepatobiliary

Heather A. Lillemoe, MD, Thomas A. Aloia, MD*

KEYWORDS

- Enhanced recovery • ERAS • Fast-track • Hepatobiliary surgery • Hepatectomy
- Pancreatectomy • Patient-reported outcomes • RIOT

KEY POINTS

- The goal of an effective Enhanced recovery after surgery (ERAS) program is the rapid return of the patient to normal life function and in the case of patients with cancer, return to intended oncologic therapies. Strategies for achieving these goals are minimization of perioperative stress, as well as excessive fluids and narcotics.
- The foundation of ERAS lies in engagement and education of the patient and caregiver. Core components universal to all ERAS include: early oral feeding, goal-directed fluid therapy, nonnarcotic analgesia, and early ambulation.
- Outcome reporting of both objective and more subjective, patient-centered, measures is imperative to advance the field, as are compliance monitoring and auditing processes.

INTRODUCTION

Enhanced recovery after surgery (ERAS) is a multidisciplinary, evidence-based approach to perioperative management. Originally implemented in colorectal surgery, the movement to optimize the care of surgical patients has expanded to most surgical subspecialties, including hepatopancreatobiliary (HPB) surgery.[1–4] Central to the concept of ERAS is reduction of the typical physiologic neuroendocrine stress response to surgery (**Fig. 1**).[5,6] By targeting specific aspects of the preoperative, intraoperative, and postoperative care, ERAS protocols create a cohesive pathway that effectively returns patients to normal homeostasis. The major goal of the ERAS initiative is to rapidly and safely return a patient to his or her baseline function after the stress of a surgical operation.

Funding Sources: Dr H.A. Lillemoe is supported by a National Institutes of Health grant T32CA009599-29.
The authors have no financial disclosures.
Department of Surgical Oncology, The University of Texas MD Anderson Cancer Center, Houston, TX, USA
* Corresponding author. Department of Surgical Oncology, The University of Texas MD Anderson Cancer Center, 1400 Pressler Street, Unit 1484, Houston, TX 77030.
E-mail address: taaloia@mdanderson.org

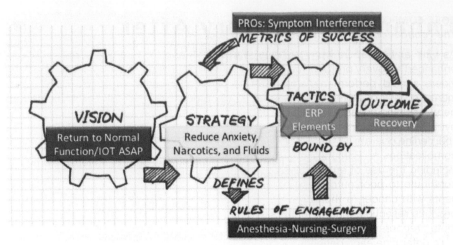

Fig. 1. The success of ERAS depends on several strategies aimed at one vision with a continuous measurement of outcomes. (*From* Manso M, Schmelz J, Aloia T. ERAS-anticipated outcomes and realistic goals. J Surg Oncol 2017;116(5):572; with permission.)

Key to enhancing patient recovery is multidisciplinary involvement and participation of all care-team members, including the patient and caregiver. The importance of patient engagement and education cannot be overemphasized, because it serves as the foundation for the entire ERAS initiative. Only with the support of the patient can the "pillars" of enhanced recovery stand. These pillars, essentially part of every ERAS pathway, are early postoperative feeding, goal-directed fluid therapy (GDFT), nonnarcotic analgesia, and early ambulation (**Fig. 2**). Of course, fundamental surgical concepts applicable to all operations continue to have relevance, including preoperative thromboembolic prophylaxis, appropriate antibiotic dosing, and the location and size of the surgical incision.

Historically, the ERAS literature has focused on outcomes such as length of stay (LOS) and complications.[7] However, the focus has begun to shift toward patient-reported outcome measures and long-term results such as return to intended oncologic therapy after oncologic resection. In addition, measures such as cost-effectiveness and compliance are emerging. Finally, it is important to recognize that ERAS is a dynamic system of care that responds and evolves as new evidence emerges.

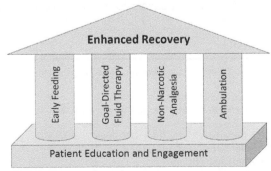

Fig. 2. The foundation and pillars of enhanced recovery after surgery. (*From* Kim BJ, Aloia TA. What is "enhanced recovery," and how can I do it? J Gastrointest Surg 2017;22(1):165; with permission.)

CORE COMPONENTS OF ENHANCED RECOVERY AFTER SURGERY
The Foundation: Patient Evaluation, Education, and Engagement

As with any preoperative evaluation, the first steps in evaluating a patient for an enhanced recovery protocol are a preoperative history and physical examination. Providers should perform a detailed review of comorbidities that may result in an increased risk of adverse outcomes after general anesthesia and hepatobiliary surgery, including advanced age, preexisting lung or heart disease, and/or signs of portal hypertension. The presence of these and other medical conditions contributing to "borderline operability" should be, when possible, optimized in an attempt to prevent complications.[8,9] Particular attention should be given to preoperative medications, including the use of anticoagulants, steroids, and narcotics, because their use may contribute to poor outcomes and challenges to ERAS implementation.[10,11] For patients with cancer, a thorough review of oncologic history including prior radiation, previous resections, intraarterial therapies, and the administration of chemotherapy (both preoperative or planned future treatment) should be described.

To determine each patient's functional status, at minimum, a validated tool such as the Eastern Cooperative Oncology Group Performance Status should be used.[12,13] With the aging population and increases in the use of potentially debilitating preoperative systemic therapy, measurement of preoperative frailty is strongly recommended.[14,15] Although the factors that define "frailty" have not been precisely defined, clinicopathologic factors such as age, preoperative albumin level, and sarcopenia have been associated with postoperative morbidity.[16–18] Objective and validated measures of functional capacity such as the Timed Up and Go Test, the 6-minute walk test, and measurement of hand grip strength can prove useful for frailty measurement.[19–21] In addition, tools such as the Mini Cog or Mini Mental Status Examination may be used to screen for neurocognitive dysfunction,[22–24] and patient-reported outcome tools are useful to determine baseline symptom burden and symptom interference.[25] Diagnosing frailty or identifying patients "at risk" via preoperative assessment does not preclude surgical intervention or participation in an ERAS pathway, but it does allow for targeted prehabilitation efforts, prediction of postoperative morbidity, and may guide modifications to multiple aspects of perioperative care.

Paramount to the concept of enhanced recovery is patient education and engagement. At the preoperative visit, the patient and his or her caregiver should be educated not only on the operation but also on the components of the ERAS protocol. Discussing the basic principles of ERAS and setting expectations substantially facilitate its successful implementation. In particular, the expectations of multimodal analgesia use, early ambulation and feeding, and timely discharge should be set. Giving each patient the team's discharge criteria is particularly effective to align patient and provider goals (**Box 1**). Hard copies of educational materials should be provided to the patient for later reference in education-level appropriate language to ensure patient understanding. As always, the patient and caregiver should be given many opportunities to ask questions regarding the operation and ERAS protocol before providing consent.

Perioperative Nutrition

The assessment of baseline nutritional status is an important component of the preoperative evaluation. A thorough workup should include questions pertaining to dietary changes and recent weight loss; body mass index (BMI); and the determination of albumin, prealbumin, and/or ferritin levels. According to the ERAS® Society guidelines for liver surgery, weight loss greater than 10% to 15% within 6 months, BMI less

> **Box 1**
> **Discharge criteria form**
>
> *Medical Criteria*
>
> - Independent ambulation
> - Adequate pain control on oral pain medicine
> - Tolerance of oral diet
> - Appropriate return of bowel function
> - No signs or symptoms of infection
> - Comorbidities well controlled
>
> *Safety/Satisfaction Criteria*
>
> - Psychologically ready for discharge
> - Safe environment/transportation
> - Demonstrate comfort with outpatient venous thromboembolic prophylaxis administration
> - Verbalize discharge instructions
> - Verbalize whom to contact for concerns
> - Confirm follow-up visit

than 18.5 kg/m^2, and serum albumin less than 3 g/dL are criteria that merit delay in surgical resection for optimization with supplemental nutrition.[26] For patients undergoing oncologic resection, the receipt of neoadjuvant chemotherapy increases the risk of malnutrition and sarcopenia. Whenever possible, both sarcopenia and sarcopenic obesity should be identified and addressed in the preoperative setting to better understand and potentially intervene on the increased risk of morbidity and mortality.[14,27]

Despite accepted guidelines regarding preoperative fasting, many patients have been instructed to endure long periods of fasting before procedures requiring general anesthesia.[28] For elective procedures in patients with normal gastric function, the current American Anesthesiologist's Association guidelines recommend clear liquid fasting up to 2 hours and "light" solids up to 6 hours before operations requiring general anesthesia.[29] This is in accordance with the ERAS® Society guidelines specific to liver and pancreas surgery.[26,30] There is strong evidence to support carbohydrate loading in colorectal surgery to maximize glycogen storage and minimize insulin resistance in the postoperative period.[31] The data supporting carbohydrate loading before hepatobiliary surgery are lacking; however, it is likely beneficial and should be considered particularly before pancreaticoduodenectomy.[26,30] Oral bowel preparation, which can lead to fluid shifts and electrolyte imbalance in the perioperative period, has little evidence or rationale in HPB surgery and is not recommended.[26,30,32]

The final key nutritional aspect of ERAS is the initiation of early postoperative feeding. The literature supports early feeding and rapid diet advancement after gastrointestinal surgery and hepatobiliary surgery, in particular.[26,33–36] Patients without contraindications to oral feeding should be given clear liquids on the day of surgery with plans for advancement to a solid diet on the day following the operation. Prophylactic use of nasogastric tubes should be avoided because this can potentiate aspiration, delay diet advancement, and contribute to unnecessary delays in ambulation and subsequent discharge.[26,30] If enteric drainage is needed, early removal is recommended. Intravenous fluids should be used judiciously. Measurement of brain natriuretic peptide (BNP) levels has recently been shown to be an accurate measure of euvolemia and a more accurate guide for postoperative fluid administration.[37] Patients tolerating clear liquids ad lib rarely require supplemental fluid administration. Antiemetic prophylaxis should be administered at the discretion of the anesthesiology team to limit postoperative nausea/vomiting and promote early feeding. The use of perioperative steroids may also be considered to ameliorate the body's stress response to surgery with added antiemetic and analgesic benefits.[38,39]

Goal-Directed Fluid Therapy

The concept of intraoperative GDFT uses hemodynamic parameters, such as stroke volume variation (SVV) and/or pulse pressure variation, to guide fluid administration. This allows dynamic assessment of intravascular volume status in order to administer the appropriate amount and type of intravenous fluid at the appropriate time and to measure the hemodynamic response to bolus. Although the more conventional parameters such as urine output, mean arterial pressure, and central venous pressure are important hemodynamic factors, SVV is more accurate in predicting fluid responsiveness intraoperatively. Benefits of GDFT have been demonstrated in a recent randomized clinical trial (RCT) comparing traditional fluid administration with GDFT, where patients treated with GDFT had a lower incidence of postoperative complications.[40]

GDFT principles should carry into the immediate postoperative period, transitioning to the use of trends in urine output and hemodynamic indices to guide resuscitation. In addition, BNP measurement is an important metric that can assist in accurate assessment of intravascular volume status postoperatively. BNP is a 32-amino acid protein produced by the cardiac myocytes in response to dilation in the setting of volume overload. It has been shown to assess intravascular volume status better than changes in blood urea nitrogen/creatinine ratio immediately after pancreatectomy.[41] More recently, a postoperative BNP-guided protocol developed at MD Anderson Cancer Center that includes daily postoperative measurement of BNP levels has been shown to reduce both cardiopulmonary and renal complications after liver surgery **(Table 1)**.[37]

Nonnarcotic and Neuraxial Analgesia

Multimodal, nonnarcotic analgesia is a core component of enhanced recovery. Opioids are not only addictive substances causing a major public-health crisis across the nation but can also have negative effects on patient experience, function, recovery, and survival. Systemic opioids provide pain relief at the expense of side effects such as drowsiness, nausea, vomiting, xerostomia, gut dysmotility, and respiratory

Table 1		
BNP-guided resuscitation algorithm for liver surgery		
BNP Level	**Fluid Administration**	**Other Intervention Indicated**
<100 pg/mL[a]	250–500 mL bolus Continue current MIVF rate	No
100–200 pg/mL	No bolus Minimize MIVF rate	No
>200 pg/mL	Minimize MIVF rate or KVO	Consider diuresis and/or cardiac workup

Abbreviations: KVO, keep vein open; MIVF, maintenance intravenous fluid.
[a] Or urine output less than 50 mL over 2 hours.

depression. These negative side effects can lead to postoperative morbidity and prolonged hospital LOS.[42] In patients with cancer, research suggests that opioids may play a role in augmenting cancer biology by activating vascular endothelial growth factor via the mu receptor, directly stimulating cancer growth and metastasis.[43–45] Data from several studies suggest improved oncologic outcomes in patients receiving opioid-sparing analgesic regimens.[46–49]

ERAS protocols are most effective when they use a multimodal opioid-sparing analgesia strategy. Preventative regimens are often used and can consist of preoperative administration of nonnarcotic neuromodulators (such as pregabalin), in combination with antiinflammatory nonsteroidal drugs (COX-2 inhibitors) and nonaddicting opiatelike substances (such as tramadol). There is also strong support for the use of regional analgesia via neuraxial or field blocks covering the incisional area. Epidural placement and other regional blocks should be performed by an experienced practitioner to cover the desired area of incision. Decision-making around these strategies requires continual communication between surgical and anesthesiology teams. The goal of preemptive strategies is to blunt the acute pain of surgical injury, typically lasting ~48 hours so that bolus narcotic dosing can be avoided. An RCT of 140 patients undergoing hepatobiliary surgery at MD Anderson Cancer Center directly compared thoracic epidural analgesia (TEA) with patient-controlled intravenous analgesia (PCA), and TEA resulted in markedly less narcotic use, lower pain scores, and superior patient-reported outcomes.[50] Additional studies have also demonstrated the oncologic benefits of these strategies.[47,49]

Some concerns surround TEA use in regards to analgesia-related complications, such as hypotension and hypoperfusion. Importantly, the aforementioned trial demonstrated comparable perioperative morbidity without an increase in analgesia-related complications in the TEA group compared with PCA group.[50] Previous data have also shown TEA leads to decreased incidence of postoperative ileus, decreased risk of postoperative pneumonia, and decreased insulin resistance.[51–53] An alternative and commonly practiced technique for regional analgesia is a transversus abdominis plane block (TAP block), where local anesthetic is injected under ultrasound guidance within the space between the internal oblique and transversus abdominis. When compared with placebo, TAP block leads to a decrease in narcotic use, lower pain scores, and a decrease in postoperative nausea and vomiting, while avoiding the need for an external delivery catheter.[54,55] The question of superiority of TEA versus TAP block for open HPB surgery remains unanswered, with current comparisons of the 2 modalities in various types of abdominal surgery showing mixed results.[56,57]

Early Ambulation and Early Removal of Tubes/Drains

Postoperative mobilization, another key aspect of ERAS, should be initiated early after surgery. Although it is a simple intervention, early ambulation can have profound effects on reducing ileus, improving pulmonary function, and decreasing postoperative thromboembolic events.[26,30] For patients with baseline functional deficits, physical and occupational therapists should be involved early in the postoperative period. Limited placement and early removal of any unnecessary drains, tubes, or catheters are helpful in facilitating this aspect of ERAS. Urinary catheters can be essential in the immediate postoperative period for hemodynamic monitoring and GDFT but should be removed as soon as patients are ambulatory (typically postoperative day 1–2). For older men, prophylactic alpha blockade can be used to avoid urinary retention and subsequent catheter replacement.

Minimally Invasive Approaches to Hepatobiliary Surgery

Experience from specialized, high-volume centers indicates that minimally invasive hepatobiliary surgery is safe and effective.[58–61] Laparoscopic liver resection (LLR) approaches have been readily adopted and are becoming standard practice for minor liver resections, particularly in the case of left lateral sectionectomies.[62] In 2009, a large multicenter study demonstrated both feasibility and safety of major laparoscopic liver resections.[59] This allowed for direct comparison of LLR procedures with those performed via open surgical approach, which highlighted important benefits of small incisions: less pain, decreased postoperative ileus, and lower hernia rates. Importantly, oncologic resection was not compromised by a laparoscopic approach.[63–66] Although there is evidence that ERAS pathways can hasten recovery after laparoscopic surgery compared with non-ERAS care, little evidence exists in regards to superiority of laparoscopy over laparotomy within ERAS protocols.[67,68] A recent double-blinded, multicenter RCT comparing laparoscopic versus open left lateral sectionectomy within an ERAS protocol failed to show any difference between groups in regards to recovery and was terminated early.[69] For pancreatic surgery, the most commonly performed minimally invasive operation is laparoscopic distal pancreatectomy. Laparoscopic enucleation and laparoscopic pancreaticoduodenectomy are being increasingly reported, as are laparoscopic approaches to the management of pancreatitis.[70] Research in both laparoscopic distal pancreatectomy and pancreaticoduodenectomy show favorable outcomes.[71,72] However, selection bias is inherent in these non-randomized analyses. Laparoscopic pancreatic surgery is feasible in particular clinical scenarios but largely depends on operator skill and experience.

For every case being considered for a minimally invasive approach, the safety, efficacy, and efficiency of the procedure must be taken into account. In addition, costs associated with minimally invasive techniques should be considered, because longer operative times and disposable instruments can lead to more charges in laparoscopy than in open surgery; however this may be counteracted by improvements in LOS.[60] Although the magnitude of impact of ERAS may be less in minimally invasive HPB surgery, the synergy between the perioperative care and the intraoperative approach can be substantial.

OUTCOMES IN HEPATOPANCREATOBILIARY AND COMPLIANCE MONITORING

Studies directly comparing enhanced recovery after HPB surgery with traditional care pathways show improvements in various metrics, namely LOS, pain-related measures, and morbidity. In a randomized trial, Jones and colleagues[1] demonstrated that ERAS resulted in more timely discharge readiness and shortened LOS compared with standard care after open liver surgery (LOS 4 vs 7 days; P<.001). Surgical complications and patient satisfaction were, however, comparable between groups. In a meta-analysis of RCTs comparing ERAS with traditional pathways for liver surgery, complications and LOS were substantially lower for patients treated by enhanced recovery.[2] A systematic review of ERAS for pancreatic surgery showed that ERAS decreased LOS and readmission rates in most studies compared with standard care. Morbidity was not found to be significantly decreased with ERAS in 5 of 6 studies, with the exception of a decrease in delayed gastric emptying with ERAS use after pancreaticoduodenectomy.[73,74] Although these results are promising, it is important to note the variation in how outcomes such as complications were measured and that ERAS criteria were not uniform across the studies.

This issue highlights the important point of compliance monitoring and auditing. ERAS® Society guidelines now exist for both liver resection and pancreaticoduodenectomy,

Table 2
The University of Texas MD Anderson Cancer Center approach to enhanced recovery in hepatobiliary surgery

	Factors	Enhanced Recovery Measures
Preoperative	Education	Procedure and ERAS-specific patient education material provided to patient and caregiver.
	Fluid Management	Saline-lock IV in preoperative holding.
	Preoperative Fasting	Clear liquids permitted up to 2 h before surgery. Solids permitted up to 6 h before surgery.
	Bowel State	No mechanical bowel preparation required.
	Preventative Analgesia	Celecoxib, 400 mg PO, pregabalin, 75 mg PO (unless age >65 y), tramadol extended release, 300 mg, PO before surgery. Anxiolytics and antiemetic medication as needed per anesthesia team.
Intraoperative	Perioperative Steroids	Dexamethasone, 10 mg, IV administration on induction of anesthesia.
	Opioid-sparing Analgesia	Acetaminophen, 1000 mg, every 6 h and minimization of narcotic use intraoperatively.
	Total Intravenous Analgesia	IV propofol as main anesthetic agent in conjunction with IV dexmedetomidine, IV ketamine, and IV lidocaine, titrated by anesthesiologist as needed.
	Fluid Management	GDFT with stroke volume monitoring.
	Regional Anesthesia	MIS: local anesthetic wound infiltration with long-acting bupivacaine. Open: epidural preferred.
	Drains	Limit use to scenarios where absolutely indicated.
Postoperative	Opioid-sparing Analgesia	Pregabalin, acetaminophen, celecoxib, and tramadol use per protocol in the postoperative period. Hydromorphone, 0.5 mg, IV every 30 min PRN breakthrough pain not relieved within 30 min of oxycodone administration. PCA only if failure of epidural.
	PRN Analgesia	Epidural titration per pain service. Nonepidural patient: mild pain, acetaminophen, 500 mg PO, every 6 h; moderate pain, tramadol, 50 mg PO, every 6 h; severe pain, hydromorphone, 0.5 mg, every 15 min x2
	Tubes and Drains	Limit use of nasogastric tubes. Early removal of foley catheter.
	Early Ambulation	Day of surgery: sit on the edge of bed; POD 1: out of bed to chair and ambulation at least 4x daily.
	Fluid Management	Hepatobiliary fluid protocol using BUN and UOP monitoring. Minimize IV fluid rate and saline lock after 600 cc PO.
	Early Oral Intake	Patients are allowed clear liquids on day of surgery. Regular diet after POD 1.
	"Ready for Discharge" Criteria	Formalized discharge criteria: independently ambulatory, pain adequately controlled (on PO medications), oral diet tolerance, appropriate return of bowel function, no signs of infection, well-controlled comorbidities.

Abbreviations: BUN, blood urea nitrogen; MIS, minimally invasive surgery; PCA, patient-controlled IV analgesia; PO, per os; POD, postoperative day; PRN, pro re nata; UOP, urine output.

creating reference lists of ERAS components stratified by grade of recommendation.[26,30] Although these guidelines are evidence-based, there is little understanding of the impact that each component has on the improvement in outcomes.[6] Similarly, without uniformity in the definition of ERAS compliance across a specialty, studies cannot be directly compared. The ERAS® Compliance Group has shown that higher compliance with ERAS protocols is associated with more substantial benefits in colorectal surgery. Thus, programs should strive not only to implement all recommended components but also to have a strategy that monitors and reports compliance.[75,76] Protocol-driven pathways are strongly recommended as a means of ensuring compliance. An example of an ERAS pathway for liver surgery in large tertiary cancer center is demonstrated in **Table 2**. The ERAS® Society has developed an auditing system, based on the guidelines, for continuous monitoring of compliance and outcomes.[5]

PATIENT-REPORTED OUTCOMES AND RETURN TO INTENDED ONCOLOGIC TREATMENT

As mentioned, the main goal of any ERAS pathway is to return the patient to his or her baseline function safely and quickly. However, functional recovery is rarely found in the medical record. Only the patient can relate their experience and their functional recovery, and validated patient-reported outcomes (PROs) are the only conduit to record these outcomes. While clinical outcomes research has shown objective improvements with ERAS compared to traditional pathways in regards to LOS, morbidity, and costs, the implementation of PROs allows for an understanding of the effect of ERAS on patient functional and emotional recovery. Validated PRO tools are now a recommended component of ERAS as they provide meaningful data to ensure that changes in practice are improving patient-centric outcomes.[77,78]

A corollary outcome that holistically captures true functional recovery in surgical oncology patients is return to intended oncologic therapy (RIOT).[79] This quality metric represents the number of patients who initiate postoperative adjuvant treatment of any kind divided by the number of patients intended to receive adjuvant therapy.[6,79] Successful tumor resection is a critical piece of oncologic care, but with high rates of multi-disciplinary management of cancer, adjuvant therapies are often recommended.[79,80] RIOT is an important outcome that can be used to validate the degree of successful recovery. Once a patient has been cleared to resume further oncologic therapy, he or she has crossed a recovery threshold that can have true survival impact. At MD Anderson Cancer Center, the implementation of an ERAS protocol after liver surgery resulted in increased RIOT rates to 95% at 21 days (compared to 87% at 32 days for standard care).[77]

SUMMARY

ERAS protocols in hepatobiliary surgery are proven to improve outcomes such as LOS and postoperative complications. Recently, a shift toward analysis of long-term oncologic and patient-centered functional outcomes suggests the superiority in ERAS in these domains compared to traditional recovery, as well. Implementation strategies, compliance measurement and outcomes feedback have the potential to further the efficacy of ERAS in HPB Surgery.

REFERENCES

1. Jones C, Kelliher L, Dickinson M, et al. Randomized clinical trial on enhanced recovery versus standard care following open liver resection. Br J Surg 2013; 100(8):1015–24.

2. Ni TG, Yang HT, Zhang H, et al. Enhanced recovery after surgery programs in patients undergoing hepatectomy: a meta-analysis. World J Gastroenterol 2015; 21(30):9209–16.
3. Barton JG. Enhanced recovery pathways in pancreatic surgery. Surg Clin North Am 2016;96(6):1301–12.
4. Page AJ, Ejaz A, Spolverato G, et al. Enhanced recovery after surgery protocols for open hepatectomy—physiology, immunomodulation, and implementation. J Gastrointest Surg 2015;19(2):387–99.
5. Ljungqvist O, Scott M, Fearon KC. Enhanced recovery after surgery: a review. JAMA Surg 2017;152(3):292–8.
6. Manso M, Schmelz J, Aloia T. ERAS-anticipated outcomes and realistic goals. J Surg Oncol 2017;116(5):570–7.
7. Day RW, Fielder S, Calhoun J, et al. Incomplete reporting of enhanced recovery elements and its impact on achieving quality improvement. Br J Surg 2015; 102(13):1594–602.
8. Kim BJ, Tzeng CD, Cooper AB, et al. Borderline operability in hepatectomy patients is associated with higher rates of failure to rescue after severe complications. J Surg Oncol 2017;115(3):337–43.
9. Tzeng CW, Katz MH, Fleming JB, et al. Morbidity and mortality after pancreaticoduodenectomy in patients with borderline resectable type C clinical classification. J Gastrointest Surg 2014;18(1):146–55 [discussion: 155–6].
10. Kim Y, Cortez AR, Wima K, et al. Impact of preoperative opioid use after emergency general surgery. J Gastrointest Surg 2018;22(6):1098–103.
11. Li Y, Stocchi L, Cherla D, et al. Association of preoperative narcotic use with postoperative complications and prolonged length of hospital stay in patients with crohn disease. JAMA Surg 2016;151(8):726–34.
12. Oken MM, Creech RH, Tormey DC, et al. Toxicity and response criteria of the Eastern Cooperative Oncology Group. Am J Clin Oncol 1982;5(6):649–55.
13. Yates JW, Chalmer B, McKegney FP. Evaluation of patients with advanced cancer using the Karnofsky performance status. Cancer 1980;45(8):2220–4.
14. Wagner D, DeMarco MM, Amini N, et al. Role of frailty and sarcopenia in predicting outcomes among patients undergoing gastrointestinal surgery. World J Gastrointest Surg 2016;8(1):27–40.
15. Beckert AK, Huisingh-Scheetz M, Thompson K, et al. Screening for frailty in thoracic surgical patients. Ann Thorac Surg 2017;103(3):956–61.
16. Reddy SK, Barbas AS, Turley RS, et al. Major liver resection in elderly patients: a multi-institutional analysis. J Am Coll Surg 2011;212(5):787–95.
17. Giovannini I, Chiarla C, Giuliante F, et al. The relationship between albumin, other plasma proteins and variables, and age in the acute phase response after liver resection in man. Amino Acids 2006;31(4):463–9.
18. Valero V 3rd, Amini N, Spolverato G, et al. Sarcopenia adversely impacts postoperative complications following resection or transplantation in patients with primary liver tumors. J Gastrointest Surg 2015;19(2):272–81.
19. Carey EJ, Steidley DE, Aqel BA, et al. Six-minute walk distance predicts mortality in liver transplant candidates. Liver Transpl 2010;16(12):1373–8.
20. Hofheinz M, Mibs M. The prognostic validity of the timed up and go test with a dual task for predicting the risk of falls in the elderly. Gerontol Geriatr Med 2016;2. 2333721416637798.
21. Partridge JS, Fuller M, Harari D, et al. Frailty and poor functional status are common in arterial vascular surgical patients and affect postoperative outcomes. Int J Surg 2015;18:57–63.

22. Korc-Grodzicki B, Sun SW, Zhou Q, et al. Geriatric assessment as a predictor of delirium and other outcomes in elderly patients with cancer. Ann Surg 2015; 261(6):1085–90.

23. Robinson TN, Wu DS, Pointer LF, et al. Preoperative cognitive dysfunction is related to adverse postoperative outcomes in the elderly. J Am Coll Surg 2012; 215(1):12–7 [discussion: 17–8].

24. Folstein MF, Folstein SE, McHugh PR. "Mini-mental state". A practical method for grading the cognitive state of patients for the clinician. J Psychiatr Res 1975; 12(3):189–98.

25. Cleeland CS, Mendoza TR, Wang XS, et al. Assessing symptom distress in cancer patients: the M.D. Anderson Symptom Inventory. Cancer 2000;89(7): 1634–46.

26. Melloul E, Hubner M, Scott M, et al. Guidelines for perioperative care for liver surgery: Enhanced Recovery After Surgery (ERAS) society recommendations. World J Surg 2016;40(10):2425–40.

27. Shen Y, Hao Q, Zhou J, et al. The impact of frailty and sarcopenia on postoperative outcomes in older patients undergoing gastrectomy surgery: a systematic review and meta-analysis. BMC Geriatr 2017;17:188.

28. Brady M, Kinn S, Stuart P. Preoperative fasting for adults to prevent perioperative complications. Cochrane Database Syst Rev 2003;(4):CD004423.

29. Practice guidelines for preoperative fasting and the use of pharmacologic agents to reduce the risk of pulmonary aspiration: application to healthy patients undergoing elective proceduresan updated report by the American Society of Anesthesiologists Task Force on preoperative fasting and the use of pharmacologic agents to reduce the risk of pulmonary aspiration*. Anesthesiology 2017; 126(3):376–93.

30. Lassen K, Coolsen MM, Slim K, et al. Guidelines for perioperative care for pancreaticoduodenectomy: Enhanced Recovery After Surgery (ERAS(R)) society recommendations. Clin Nutr 2012;31(6):817–30.

31. Gustafsson UO, Scott MJ, Schwenk W, et al. Guidelines for perioperative care in elective colonic surgery: Enhanced Recovery After Surgery (ERAS((R))) Society recommendations. World J Surg 2013;37(2):259–84.

32. Lavu H, Kennedy EP, Mazo R, et al. Preoperative mechanical bowel preparation does not offer a benefit for patients who undergo pancreaticoduodenectomy. Surgery 2010;148(2):278–84.

33. Lassen K, Kjaeve J, Fetveit T, et al. Allowing normal food at will after major upper gastrointestinal surgery does not increase morbidity: a randomized multicenter trial. Ann Surg 2008;247(5):721–9.

34. Hwang SE, Jung MJ, Cho BH, et al. Clinical feasibility and nutritional effects of early oral feeding after pancreaticoduodenectomy. Korean J Hepatobiliary Pancreat Surg 2014;18(3):84–9.

35. Han-Geurts IJ, Hop WC, Kok NF, et al. Randomized clinical trial of the impact of early enteral feeding on postoperative ileus and recovery. Br J Surg 2007;94(5): 555–61.

36. Warner SG, Jutric Z, Nisimova L, et al. Early recovery pathway for hepatectomy: data-driven liver resection care and recovery. Hepatobiliary Surg Nutr 2017;6(5): 297–311.

37. Patel SH, Kim BJ, Tzeng CD, et al. Reduction of cardiopulmonary/renal complications with serum bnp-guided volume status management in posthepatectomy patients. J Gastrointest Surg 2018;22(3):467–76.

38. Richardson AJ, Laurence JM, Lam VWT. Use of pre-operative steroids in liver resection: a systematic review and meta-analysis. HPB (Oxford) 2014;16(1):12–9.
39. Waldron NH, Jones CA, Gan TJ, et al. Impact of perioperative dexamethasone on postoperative analgesia and side-effects: systematic review and meta-analysis. Br J Anaesth 2013;110(2):191–200.
40. Correa-Gallego C, Tan KS, Arslan-Carlon V, et al. Goal-directed fluid therapy using stroke volume variation for resuscitation after low central venous pressure assisted liver resection. a randomized clinical trial. J Am Coll Surg 2015;221(2): 591–601.
41. Berri RN, Sahai SK, Durand JB, et al. Serum brain naturietic peptide measurements reflect fluid balance after pancreatectomy. J Am Coll Surg 2012;214(5): 778–87.
42. Kehlet H. Postoperative opioid sparing to hasten recovery: what are the issues? Anesthesiology 2005;102(6):1083–5.
43. Lennon FE, Moss J, Singleton PA. The mu-opioid receptor in cancer progression: is there a direct effect? Anesthesiology 2012;116(4):940–5.
44. Lennon FE, Mirzapoiazova T, Mambetsariev B, et al. The Mu opioid receptor promotes opioid and growth factor-induced proliferation, migration and Epithelial Mesenchymal Transition (EMT) in human lung cancer. PLoS One 2014;9(3): e91577.
45. Gupta K, Kshirsagar S, Chang L, et al. Morphine stimulates angiogenesis by activating proangiogenic and survival-promoting signaling and promotes breast tumor growth. Cancer Res 2002;62(15):4491–8.
46. Biki B, Mascha E, Moriarty DC, et al. Anesthetic technique for radical prostatectomy surgery affects cancer recurrence: a retrospective analysis. Anesthesiology 2008;109(2):180–7.
47. Exadaktylos AK, Buggy DJ, Moriarty DC, et al. Can anesthetic technique for primary breast cancer surgery affect recurrence or metastasis? Anesthesiology 2006;105(4):660–4.
48. Wang K, Qu X, Wang Y, et al. Effect of mu agonists on long-term survival and recurrence in nonsmall cell lung cancer patients. Medicine 2015;94(33):e1333.
49. Zimmitti G, Soliz J, Aloia TA, et al. Positive impact of epidural analgesia on oncologic outcomes in patients undergoing resection of colorectal liver metastases. Ann Surg Oncol 2016;23(3):1003–11.
50. Aloia TA, Kim BJ, Segraves-Chun YS, et al. A randomized controlled trial of postoperative thoracic epidural analgesia versus intravenous patient-controlled analgesia after major hepatopancreatobiliary surgery. Ann Surg 2017;266(3):545–54.
51. Jorgensen H, Wetterslev J, Moiniche S, et al. Epidural local anaesthetics versus opioid-based analgesic regimens on postoperative gastrointestinal paralysis, PONV and pain after abdominal surgery. Cochrane Database Syst Rev 2000;(4):CD001893.
52. Popping DM, Elia N, Marret E, et al. Protective effects of epidural analgesia on pulmonary complications after abdominal and thoracic surgery: a meta-analysis. Arch Surg 2008;143(10):990–9 [discussion: 1000].
53. Uchida I, Asoh T, Shirasaka C, et al. Effect of epidural analgesia on postoperative insulin resistance as evaluated by insulin clamp technique. Br J Surg 1988;75(6): 557–62.
54. Johns N, O'Neill S, Ventham NT, et al. Clinical effectiveness of transversus abdominis plane (TAP) block in abdominal surgery: a systematic review and meta-analysis. Colorectal Dis 2012;14(10):e635–42.

55. De Oliveira GS Jr, Castro-Alves LJ, Nader A, et al. Transversus abdominis plane block to ameliorate postoperative pain outcomes after laparoscopic surgery: a meta-analysis of randomized controlled trials. Anesth Analg 2014;118(2):454–63.

56. Niraj G, Kelkar A, Jeyapalan I, et al. Comparison of analgesic efficacy of subcostal transversus abdominis plane blocks with epidural analgesia following upper abdominal surgery. Anaesthesia 2011;66(6):465–71.

57. Pirrera B, Alagna V, Lucchi A, et al. Transversus abdominis plane (TAP) block versus thoracic epidural analgesia (TEA) in laparoscopic colon surgery in the ERAS program. Surg Endosc 2018;32(1):376–82.

58. Koffron AJ, Auffenberg G, Kung R, et al. Evaluation of 300 minimally invasive liver resections at a single institution: less is more. Ann Surg 2007;246(3):385–92 [discussion: 392–4].

59. Dagher I, O'Rourke N, Geller DA, et al. Laparoscopic major hepatectomy: an evolution in standard of care. Ann Surg 2009;250(5):856–60.

60. Buell JF, Thomas MT, Rudich S, et al. Experience with more than 500 minimally invasive hepatic procedures. Ann Surg 2008;248(3):475–86.

61. Boggi U, Amorese G, Vistoli F, et al. Laparoscopic pancreaticoduodenectomy: a systematic literature review. Surg Endosc 2015;29(1):9–23.

62. Wakabayashi G, Cherqui D, Geller DA, et al. Recommendations for laparoscopic liver resection: a report from the second international consensus conference held in Morioka. Ann Surg 2015;261(4):619–29.

63. Ito K, Ito H, Are C, et al. Laparoscopic versus open liver resection: a matched-pair case control study. J Gastrointest Surg 2009;13(12):2276–83.

64. Yin Z, Fan X, Ye H, et al. Short- and long-term outcomes after laparoscopic and open hepatectomy for hepatocellular carcinoma: a global systematic review and meta-analysis. Ann Surg Oncol 2013;20(4):1203–15.

65. Fancellu A, Rosman AS, Sanna V, et al. Meta-analysis of trials comparing minimally-invasive and open liver resections for hepatocellular carcinoma. J Surg Res 2011;171(1):e33–45.

66. Parks KR, Kuo YH, Davis JM, et al. Laparoscopic versus open liver resection: a meta-analysis of long-term outcome. HPB (Oxford) 2014;16(2):109–18.

67. Ratti F, Cipriani F, Reineke R, et al. Impact of ERAS approach and minimally-invasive techniques on outcome of patients undergoing liver surgery for hepatocellular carcinoma. Dig Liver Dis 2016;48(10):1243–8.

68. Liang X, Ying H, Wang H, et al. Enhanced recovery care versus traditional care after laparoscopic liver resections: a randomized controlled trial. Surg Endosc 2018;32(6):2746–57.

69. Wong-Lun-Hing EM, van Dam RM, van Breukelen GJ, et al. Randomized clinical trial of open versus laparoscopic left lateral hepatic sectionectomy within an enhanced recovery after surgery programme (ORANGE II study). Br J Surg 2017;104(5):525–35.

70. Niess H, Werner J. Indications and contraindications for laparoscopic pancreas surgery. In: Conrad C, Gayet B, editors. Laparoscopic liver, pancreas, and biliary surgery. 1st edition. New York: John Wiley & Sons, Ltd; 2017. p. 337–48.

71. Kooby DA, Hawkins WG, Schmidt CM, et al. A multicenter analysis of distal pancreatectomy for adenocarcinoma: is laparoscopic resection appropriate? J Am Coll Surg 2010;210(5):779–85, 786–77.

72. Correa-Gallego C, Dinkelspiel HE, Sulimanoff I, et al. Minimally-invasive vs open pancreaticoduodenectomy: systematic review and meta-analysis. J Am Coll Surg 2014;218(1):129–39.

73. Kagedan DJ, Ahmed M, Devitt KS, et al. Enhanced recovery after pancreatic surgery: a systematic review of the evidence. HPB (Oxford) 2015;17(1):11–6.
74. Balzano G, Zerbi A, Braga M, et al. Fast-track recovery programme after pancreatico- duodenectomy reduces delayed gastric emptying. Br J Surg 2008; 95(11):1387–93.
75. Li L, Jin J, Min S, et al. Compliance with the enhanced recovery after surgery protocol and prognosis after colorectal cancer surgery: a prospective cohort study. Oncotarget 2017;8(32):53531–41.
76. ERAS Compliance Group. The impact of enhanced recovery protocol compliance on elective colorectal cancer resection: results from an international registry. Ann Surg 2015;261(6):1153–9.
77. Day RW, Cleeland CS, Wang XS, et al. Patient-reported outcomes accurately measure the value of an enhanced recovery program in liver surgery. J Am Coll Surg 2015;221(6):1023–30.e1-2.
78. Abola RE, Bennett-Guerrero E, Kent ML, et al. American Society for Enhanced Recovery and perioperative quality initiative joint consensus statement on patient-reported outcomes in an enhanced recovery pathway. Anesth Analg 2018;126(6):1874–82.
79. Aloia TA, Zimmitti G, Conrad C, et al. Return to intended oncologic treatment (RIOT): a novel metric for evaluating the quality of oncosurgical therapy for malignancy. J Surg Oncol 2014;110(2):107–14.
80. Tzeng C-WD, Cao HST, Lee JE, et al. Treatment sequencing for resectable pancreatic cancer: influence of early metastases and surgical complications on multimodality therapy completion and survival. J Gastrointest Surg 2014;18(1): 16–25.

Enhanced Recovery After Surgery: Urology

Ava Saidian, MD, Jeffrey Wells Nix, MD*

KEYWORDS

- ERAS • Enhanced recovery after surgery • Clinical care pathways
- Perioperative care

KEY POINTS

- Evidence-based perioperative care pathways seek to improve patient recovery through thoughtful standardization of perioperative care.
- Evidence-based perioperative care pathways in urology began with efforts to reduce length of stay (LOS) for radical prostatectomy patients and have expanded to partial nephrectomy and radical cystectomy.
- Significant LOS reductions have been shown for these major procedures through these standardized care pathways.
- Future research is needed in urology for the cost-effectiveness of these protocols, in both inpatient costs and the outpatient economic impact of faster, more efficient patient recovery.

INTRODUCTION

Enhanced recovery after surgery (ERAS) programs were developed as a type of standardized evidence-based perioperative care protocols. The necessity and benefit of clinical care pathways is not a new phenomenon in urology. In the early to mid 90s, radical retropubic prostatectomy (RRP) for prostate cancer was often a procedure with an average inpatient length of stay (LOS) around 6 days in the United States.[1] Efforts to improve perioperative care at that time was often centered around reducing cost by decreasing LOS, because this was one of the main drivers of cost for both healthy and sick patients. In 1994 the group from Vanderbilt published their experience with a collaborative care pathway in open prostatectomy for patients with prostate cancer, which significantly decreased their mean LOS (5.7–3.6 days) without an increase in perioperative complications. They subsequently further honed ERAS to achieve discharge of more than 90% of open postprostatectomy patients by postoperative day (POD) 3.[2] The components of their pathways were progressive for the time, however, what is now considered many of the basic tenets of ERAS (eg, multimodal

Disclosure Statement: The authors have nothing to disclose.
Department Urology, University of Alabama at Birmingham, 1720 2nd Avenue South, Birmingham, AL 35294, USA
* Corresponding author.
E-mail address: jnix@uabmc.edu

anesthesia, early ambulation, early diet initiation, etc.). Surveillance, Epidemiology, and End Results (SEER) data demonstrated similar findings throughout the country with decrease in hospital stay of around 3 days when comparing patients from early 90s with early 2000s for open prostatectomy.[3] This trend continued to evolve as the advent of minimally invasive prostatectomy (MIP) occurred during the ensuing decade. In 2002, using the Nationwide Inpatient Sample (NIS), it was estimated that 1.4% of prostatectomies were MIP with an increase to more than 40% in 2008. In that time period the inpatient LOS decreased significantly for both MIP and open prostatectomy to less than 2 days in many centers, as ERAS pathways diffused across institutions regardless of surgical approach.[4] These ERAS pathways began to include, in addition to those previously mentioned, even more key modern components such as omission of oral bowel preparation, limited exposure to narcotics, and scheduled Ketorolac.[5]

Even though RRP was an initial impetus for ERAS pathways in urologic oncology, most of the efforts in more recent years has focused on radical cystectomy for bladder cancer. For patients with muscle invasive bladder cancer or high-risk nonmuscle invasive bladder cancer, radical cystectomy (RC) with pelvic lymph node dissection (PLND) is the gold standard of treatment. RC for bladder cancer is a perfect case study for ERAS pathways. It is a complex procedure with high perioperative complication rate in an older patient population with more medical comorbid conditions and a high clinical cost. The annual cost estimates for bladder cancer in 2010 was close to $4 billion with an estimated increase to more than $5 billion by 2020. Bladder cancer has the highest total Medicare payment cost per patient from diagnosis to death, with a large percentage of that cost attributable to complications of treatment.[6] Early efforts to advance perioperative care around ERAS elements for cystectomy began in 2002 and 2003 at key centers of excellence. Pruthi and colleagues[7] used a fast track program of early diet initiation, immediate nasogastric (NG) tube removal, and gum chewing to achieve a mean LOS of 5.0 days. In comparison, NIS data from 2006 to 2014 showed average 10.7 LOS for cystectomy in the United States.[8] Overall outcomes are still in need of improvement across the field for cystectomy patients. Using NSQIP data from 2010 to 2015 of more than 6500 RC procedures the average LOS was still 9.2 days and readmission rate was 21.4%.[9]

ERAS shares many elements that are relevant to major procedures across a multitude of surgical disciplines including urology. The ERAS components that apply to major urologic procedures are in general not procedure specific; however, some key components will have different application in certain procedures. It was the investigators' intent to describe the overall implementation of these elements in urology with unique elements including where relevant (**Table 1**).

Preoperative Items

Patient education and counseling

Comprehensive counseling of patients and their families has been shown to improve recovery and reduce complications after surgery. This should include both verbal and written information that includes the specifics of the ERAS pathway, hospital stay, discharge plan, and anesthesia plan. Comprehensive education and counseling can reduce surgical anxiety and potentially decrease the recovery period around surgery.[6] Preoperative education is a key component in regards to RC and urinary diversion, because misunderstandings about urinary diversion can have a negative impact on patient quality of life and their postoperative course leading to delays in discharge.[6] The American Urological Association and the Wound Ostomy Continence Nurse Society released a joint statement recommending that patients with the creation of a urostomy, as a possible outcome of a procedure, should have stoma marking done

Table 1
Urology ERAS elements

	ERAS Item	Unique Application to Urologic Surgery
PREOP Items	Patient Education and Counseling	Detailed counseling about urinary diversion and expectations
	Patient Selection and Optimization	Most of the cystectomy patients are malnourished to some degree
	Oral Bowel Preparation	• No benefit to oral bowel prep in cystectomy patients • No high-level evidence for prostatectomy patients
	Preoperative Fasting and Carbohydrate Load	N/A
	Alvimopan Administration	Earlier first bowel movement, shorter LOS, and decreased incidence of ileus in cystectomy patients
	Pre-anesthesia Medications	N/A
INTRAOP Items	Antibiotic Recommendations	• Clean-contaminated procedure; recommend second- or third- generation cephalosporin
	Anesthesia Considerations	N/A
	Surgical Approach	Decreased LOS in robotic approach compared with open
	Perioperative Fluid Management	GDFT in RC patients show decreased incidence of ileus and post-op nausea and vomiting
	Intraoperative Hypothermia Prevention	N/A
	Resection Site Drainage	Peritoneal drainage is not necessary in patients undergoing RARP, even with extended PLND
POSTOP Items	NG Tube	Routine NG tube removal after RC surgery
	Urinary Drainage	• In RP patients, cystogram should be considered before catheter removal or longer catheter times in patients with high risk of urinary anastomotic leakage • May be some short-term benefits of SP vs UC; however no long-term functional differences • Neobladder: recommend frequent irrigation of any newly formed neobladder. No official recommendations for catheter during after surgery; however most recommend 2 wk minimum
	Early Ambulation	Early ambulation can decrease thromboembolic events, pulmonary complications, and ileus risk
	Early Diet Initiation	No specific studies in urologic surgery
	Postoperative Pain Management	Opioid sparing protocols and alvimopan have been shown to reduce LOS in RC patients

in the preoperative setting by an experienced, education clinician. If at all possible this should be a provider with specific training in ostomy site selection.[10]

Patient selection and medical optimization

All patients benefit from preoperative medical optimization. This often includes diet and exercise regimen, optimization of health conditions (eg, hypertension, diabetes), and reduction in harmful health behaviors (eg, reduction in alcohol intake and smoking cessation).[11] General perioperative guidance suggests patients should refrain from smoking for at least 8 weeks before surgery.[12]

Malnutrition is a known risk factor for surgical complications. Inadequate intake of food for more than 14 days is associated with higher mortality, higher cost, increased LOS, and increased complications in patients undergoing surgery for cancer.[13] An additional concern is evidence elucidating an increase in the rate of malnutrition in patients receiving neoadjuvant chemotherapy as part of their cancer care.[13] Nutrition screening is an important preoperative tool because many urologic surgeries involve the care of patients with cancer. Especially validated for preoperative malnutrition assessment for surgical patients, the Nutritional Risk Score, by assessing weight loss, food intake, and body mass index, is a valuable tool to define nutrition-related surgical risk.[14] Assessment can lead to intervention as well. In a randomized trial of oral nutritional supplements versus dietary advice alone in colorectal surgery patients identified as malnourished and preoperative weight loss, patients receiving oral nutritional supplements had a lower infection rate.[13]

RC patients are at increased risk for malnutrition for a myriad of reasons (increased age, multimodel neoadjuvant chemotherapy, cancer, etc.). Estimates as high as 87% of cystectomy patients are malnourished to some degree,[15] and malnutrition at the time of surgery in this patient population has been associated with increased complication rates and an independent risk factor for perioperative mortality.[16] A recent randomized control trial (RCT) did suggest a benefit to immunonutrition in RC patients for possible reduction of postoperative infections.[14]

Oral bowel preparation

Historically oral bowel preparation has been performed in patients undergoing surgery requiring bowel resection.[17] Level 1 evidence exists for the omission of routine preoperative bowel preparation before colorectal surgery. There have been 3 large studies with similar outcomes in RC with ileal conduit urinary diversion.[18,19,20] These studies have shown that there is no difference in complication rate, LOS, or time to first bowel movement with or without bowel preparation. In patients undergoing radical prostatectomy, the incidence of rectal injury overall is less than 1%. This injury can occur during the posterior dissection of the prostate or seminal vesicles. There are situations where the rate of rectal injury is higher, such as patients with prior bouts of chronic prostatitis, history of prior transurethral resection of the prostate, history of prior pelvic radiation, or with locally advanced disease.[21] Salvage prostatectomy, for the treatment of locally recurrent prostate cancer after primary therapy, most commonly radiation, had a rectal injury rate historically of 15% to 20%.[22] Most modern series have shown a rectal injury rate that is less than 5%. This rate is still higher than in the primary setting but overall very low. Experts have advised consideration of mechanical bowel preparation in these patients, but there is no high-level evidence examining the necessity.[21]

Preoperative fasting and carbohydrate load

The historical paradigm of preoperative fasting has included nothing to eat or drink for patients after midnight before surgery requiring general anesthesia. There is no evidence of an increased risk of anesthesia-related complications if patients are allowed liquids up to 2 hours before surgery and solids 6 hours.[11] In fact perioperative oral intake of a clear liquid rich in complex carbohydrates 2 to 3 hours before surgery may have beneficial effects for patients.[23]

Alvimopan administration

Alvimopan is a mu opioid antagonist that can blunt the harmful effects of narcotics on the gastrointestinal tract.[24] Alvimopan has been studied specifically in urologic patients undergoing RC and urinary diversion. In this patient population there is an RCT showing earlier first bowel movement, shorter LOS, and decreased ileus in patients taking alvimopan compared with placebo perioperative.[25]

Preanesthesia medications

Patients undergoing major urologic surgery will often be treated with anxiolytic medication as part of their anesthetic protocol. Long-acting benzodiazepines are associated with cognitive side effects in elderly patients. These agents can also impair ERAS protocols because it may delay mobilization postoperatively. ERAS® guidelines recommend short-acting anxiolytics in the setting of their use.[11]

Intraoperative Items

Antibiotic recommendations

Urologic procedures should follow the guidelines laid out by the National Surgical Infection Prevention Project, and thus antibiotics should be administered less than 1 hour before surgery and before skin incision.[9] Robot-assisted radical prostatectomy and RC as well as other urologic procedures in which the urinary tract is opened are clean-contaminated procedures; guidelines exist for a second- or third-generation cephalosporin.[11,26] The Pasadena Consensus Panel for robotic cystectomy adds that the antibiotics should be extended for 24 hours for men and 48 hours for women.[27]

Anesthesia considerations

There are no prospective trials evaluating a specific anesthetic protocol for urologic surgical patients from an ERAS perspective. Many clinical care pathways have used different analgesic techniques to decrease opioid usage.

Surgical approach

Many ERAS pathways and fast track programs for surgical recovery have been associated with minimally invasive approaches. However, there are no randomized controlled trials comparing open, lap, and robotic approaches in terms of perioperative care for urologic operations. In terms of RRP, most of these procedures are performed robotically throughout the country.

Robotic RC is a relatively new surgical technique with the first reported study showing its feasibility in 2003.[28] More recently the International Robotic Cystectomy Consortium was created to better elucidate this procedure and its risks and benefits. In 2014 experts in open and robotic RC met at the Pasadena Consensus Panel for Robotic Cystectomy to develop best practice statements for this procedure. Oncologic measures of quality such as positive margin status and lymph node yield have been found to be comparable between open and robotic approaches. LOS has been shown to be decreased in the robotic approach.[11]

Perioperative fluid management

Individualized goal-directed fluid therapy (GDFT) is a key component of ERAS pathways. Its impact is most likely felt in patients with higher ASA scores and lower thresholds for variable management; however high-quality studies in urology are lacking. In an RCT investigating fluid management in RC patients, a strategy of GDFT (in this setting via esophageal probe) resulted in decreased ileus and decreased nausea and emesis postoperatively.[29] More studies in urologic surgery are key because there are many key urologic procedures in which urine output, a key indicator of fluid status, is not available for a significant portion of the procedure because of the procedure type (eg, cystectomy, prostatectomy, urinary diversion).

Intraoperative hypothermia prevention

ERAS® society recommendations are for sound monitoring and management of patient temperatures in the operating room to maintain normothermia. There are no specific studies in urology ERAS pathways evaluating this as a singular item.[11]

Resection site drainage

A peritoneal drain is a standard practice for many surgeons performing urologic procedures such as radical prostatectomy, cystectomy, partial nephrectomy, as well as many reconstructive cases. For patients undergoing robotic prostatectomy and extended pelvic lymph node dissection (ePLND), a peritoneal drain is potentially placed in an attempt to prevent symptomatic lymphocele or urinoma formation. However, in a study of 521 patients followed closely with serial abdominal ultrasounds, after RARP with PLND the development of symptomatic lymphoceles was not common (3%). An RCT of 189 patients randomized to pelvic drain versus no pelvic drain in those undergoing RARP for prostate cancer identified no difference in adverse events between the 2 groups.[30] Most of the patients in that trial did undergo an ePLND. It is the investigators' belief that in most patients undergoing RARP with ePLND robotic prostatectomy, even with extended lymph node dissection, a peritoneal drain is not necessary.

Another common procedure where peritoneal drains have commonly been used is open partial nephrectomy or robotic partial nephrectomy for the potential of collection system injury and potential urine leak with deep tumor resections. Several studies have shown that the incidence of urine leaks in modern setting is very uncommon and routine drain placement is not necessary.[31–33]

ERAS® society guidelines for RC mention that omission of postoperative drain in the peritoneal cavity after colorectal surgery has been shown to be safe but that evidence specifically for cystectomy is lacking.[11]

Postoperative Items

Nasogastric tube management

Immediate removal of the NG tube at the end of the surgical procedure is widely used for most urologic procedures. In RC with urinary diversion, historically the NG tube would remain until return of bowel function. A trend toward early removal however emerged with increasing evidence of the lack of necessity. A Cochrane meta-analysis of 33 RCTs in patients undergoing abdominal surgery noted that prophylactic NG maintenance after surgery was not necessary and did not prevent complications.[11] The ERAS® society guidelines as well as the Pasadena Consensus Panel for robotic cystectomy recommend avoidance of routine NG tube continuation after surgery.[11,27]

Urinary drainage

Urinary drainage is an area that is especially important in urologic procedures and also a unique component of our pathways. For RRP a vesicourethral (VUR) anastomosis is performed after removal of the prostate. Historically catheters were left in for long periods of time and a cystogram was performed before catheter removal to ensure that the connection was without leakage. Most of the providers no longer perform a cystogram before catheter removal; however, there are still situations when a cystogram may provide value and it is not without controversy. A recent study by Tillier and colleagues[34] performed cystogram on all patients after prostatectomy and noted a VUR anastomosis leakage rate of 20%. This rate is consistent with that reported in previous studies ranging from 5% to 20%. They noted 15% of patients with grade 2 or 3 leakage, and noted grade 3 leakage only in 4% of patients. The interesting component of this study was that in their second cohort they continued to perform cystograms in every patient and removed the urinary catheter early, independent of leakage on the cystogram at the anastomosis. This cohort was key to highlighting risks of early catheter removal in men with VUR leakage and subsequent functional consequences. The group that had early catheter removal regardless of the cystogram findings had an increased risk for acute urinary retention, voiding complaints at 6 months after surgery, as well as need for urethrotomy, with the risk highest in those men with the worst leakage noted on cystogram (grade 2 and 3). In men without cystogram evidence of leakage there was no difference in outcomes between the 2 cohorts. The men with highest risk for VUR leakage on cystogram were those with large prostates and preexisting lower urinary tract symptoms before surgery. Further studies are needed; however, the urologist should consider cystogram before catheter removal or simply longer catheter times in patients in whome there is concern about the integrity of the anastomosis at the end of the procedure, as well as those identified as higher risk in this study (ie, larger prostate size and preexisting significant lower urinary tract symptoms).[34] The duration that the urinary catheter needs to stay in after prostatectomy is also debatable with lengths ranging from 2 days to 2 weeks. There was a recent meta-analysis that examined the role of a urethral catheter (UC) or suprapubic tube (ST) as the optimal drainage strategy after RRP. The study did not find a difference in either approach, except a statistically significant advantage for the ST in terms of bother or discomfort over the UC up to POD 7. The investigators conclude that overall there is no superior drainage but that ST may be favorable in terms of discomfort in the immediate post-op period.[35] More importantly there did not seem to be a difference when evaluating drainage type with longer-term functional outcomes.

RC with orthotopic neobladder also requires the placement of a UC after surgery. There are no studies evaluating in a prospective randomized fashion the best time for removal of this catheter. The Pasadena Consensus Panel for best practices in robotic assisted RC suggests that frequent irrigation of a newly formed neobladder (starting the night of surgery) is needed in order to remove mucus.[27] An EAU working group on ERAS for robotic cystectomy could not come to a consensus in terms of best timing for UC removal in these patients; however, 70% of the committee stated that they would leave the catheter in for a minimum of 14 days.[15]

Early ambulation
As is true in most ERAS pathways there are no specific studies in urology evaluating early mobility in general or with specific interventions in an isolated fashion. However, early mobilization can potentially decrease thromboembolic events and pulmonary complications as well as ileus risk and therefore is common practice in urologic ERAS pathways.[11]

Early diet initiation
This has been a mainstay component in many of the early ERAS pathways in urology. There have been no studies showing a direct relationship to early diet initiation and a particular outcome in urologic surgery, because this is often one of several components of an ERAS pathway. However, in a meta-analysis of major abdominal surgery early diet initiation was associated with lower perioperative morbidity and mortality.[14] Diet initiation should be enteral, because parenteral nutrition has significant

associated costs, risks, and no benefit in patients for whom a period of diet interruption is less than 7 days.[16]

Postoperative pain management

It is important in any ERAS pathway to minimize opioid usage and its resultant detriments to recovery. Opioid sparing protocols in urology have used anesthetic adjuncts such as epidural catheters, intrathecal, regional blocks, intravenous lidocaine, ketamine, continuous infusion of local anesthesia via catheters directed near the wound, as well as others to limit immediate post-op pain and thus the need for opioids. The incorporation of these adjuncts and incorporation of alvimopan have been key drivers to reduce LOS associated with RC.

SUMMARY

The big drivers for ERAS pathways in the future will continue to be improving perioperative care for patients but also driving down cost through standardization and complication reduction. These protocols require significant collaboration from surgeons and anesthesiologists. Future protocols in urology could include attempts to convert RARP and robotic partial nephrectomy from a 1-night stay to an outpatient procedure to continue to reduce cost and improve recovery rates. RC continues to require further research as much of the data are extrapolated from colorectal surgery. This procedure is still associated with a high complication rate in an older, sicker patient population. Further research into the downstream economic impact of quicker, more efficient recovery is also a key part of the future of these studies.

REFERENCES

1. Koch MO, Smith JA, Hodge EM, et al. Prospective development of a cost-efficient program for radical retropubic prostatectomy. Urology 1994;44:311–8.
2. Chang SS, Cole E, Smith JA, et al. Safely reducing length of stay after open radical retropubic prostatectomy under the guidance of a clinical care pathway. Cancer 2005;104:747–51.
3. Jacobs BL, Zhang Y, Tan H-J, et al. Hospitalization trends after prostate and bladder surgery: implications of potential payment reforms. J Urol 2013;189:59–65.
4. Hofer MD, Meeks JJ, Cashy J, et al. Impact of increasing prevalence of minimally invasive prostatectomy on open prostatectomy observed in the national inpatient sample and national surgical quality improvement program. J Endourol 2013;27: 102–7.
5. Nelson B, Kaufman M, Broughton G, et al. Comparison of length of hospital stay between radical retropubic prostatectomy and robotic assisted laparoscopic prostatectomy. J Urol 2007;177:929–31.
6. Maloney I, Parker DC, Cookson MS, et al. Bladder cancer recovery pathways: a systematic review. Bladder Cancer 2017;3:269–81.
7. Pruthi RS, Nielsen M, Smith A, et al. Fast track program in patients undergoing radical cystectomy: results in 362 consecutive patients. J Am Coll Surg 2010; 210:93–9.
8. Groeben C, Koch R, Baunacke M, et al. Urinary diversion after radical cystectomy for bladder cancer: comparing trends in the US and Germany from 2006 to 2014. Ann Surg Oncol 2018;66:156–8.
9. Johnson SC, Smith ZL, Golan S, et al. Temporal trends in perioperative morbidity for radical cystectomy using the National Surgical Quality Improvement Program database. Urol Oncol 2017;35:659.e13–9.

10. bdryden. WOCN Society and ASCRS position statement. 2015. p. 1–10.
11. Cerantola Y, Valerio M, Persson B, et al. Guidelines for perioperative care after radical cystectomy for bladder cancer: ERAS society recommendations. Clin Nutr 2013;32:879–87.
12. Thomsen T, Villebro N, Møller AM. Interventions for preoperative smoking cessation. Edited byCochrane Tobacco Addiction Group. Cochrane Database Syst Rev 2014;(120):CD002294.
13. Sandrucci S, Beets G, Braga M, et al. Perioperative nutrition and enhanced recovery after surgery in gastrointestinal cancer patients. A position paper by the ESSO task force in collaboration with the ERAS society (ERAS coalition). Eur J Surg Oncol 2018;44(4):509–14.
14. Zainfeld D, Djaladat H. Enhanced recovery after urologic surgery-Current applications and future directions. Edited byCR Schmidt. J Surg Oncol 2017;116:630–7.
15. Collins JW, Patel H, Adding C, et al. Enhanced recovery after robot-assisted radical cystectomy: EAU Robotic Urology Section Scientific Working Group Consensus View. Eur Urol 2016;70:649–60.
16. Cerantola Y, Valerio M, Hubner M, et al. Are patients at nutritional risk more prone to complications after major urological surgery? J Urol 2013;190:2126–32.
17. Rollins KE, Javanmard-Emamghissi H, Lobo DN. Impact of mechanical bowel preparation in elective colorectal surgery: a meta-analysis. World J Gastroenterol 2018;24:519–36.
18. Hashad MME, Atta M, Elabbady A, et al. Safety of no bowel preparation before ileal urinary diversion. BJU Int 2012;110:E1109–13.
19. Large MC, Kiriluk KJ, DeCastro GJ, et al. The impact of mechanical bowel preparation on postoperative complications for patients undergoing cystectomy and urinary diversion. J Urol 2012;188:1801–5.
20. Xu R, Zhao X, Zhong Z, et al. No advantage is gained by preoperative bowel preparation in radical cystectomy and ileal conduit: a randomized controlled trial of 86 patients. Int Urol Nephrol 2010;42:947–50.
21. Taneja SS, Shah O. Complications of urologic surgery. New York: Elsevier; 2017.
22. Russo P. Salvage radical prostatectomy after radiation therapy and brachytherapy. J Endourol 2000;14:385–90.
23. Sarin A, Chen L-L, Wick EC. Enhanced recovery after surgery-Preoperative fasting and glucose loading-A review. Edited byCR Schmidt. J Surg Oncol 2017;116:578–82.
24. Delaney CP, Craver C, Gibbons MM, et al. Evaluation of clinical outcomes with alvimopan in clinical practice. Ann Surg 2012;255:731–8.
25. Lee CT, Chang SS, Kamat AM, et al. Alvimopan accelerates gastrointestinal recovery after radical cystectomy: a multicenter randomized placebo-controlled trial. Eur Urol 2014;66:265–72.
26. Montorsi F, Wilson TG, Rosen RC, et al. Best practices in robot-assisted radical prostatectomy: recommendations of the pasadena consensus panel. Eur Urol 2012;62:368–81.
27. Wilson TG, Guru K, Rosen RC, et al. Best practices in robot-assisted radical cystectomy and urinary reconstruction: recommendations of the pasadena consensus panel. Eur Urol 2015;67:363–75.
28. Jeong W, Kumar R, Menon M. Past, present and future of urological robotic surgery. Investig Clin Urol 2016;57:75–83.
29. Pillai P, McEleavy I, Gaughan M, et al. A double-blind randomized controlled clinical trial to assess the effect of Doppler optimized intraoperative fluid management on outcome following radical cystectomy. J Urol 2011;186:2201–6.

30. Chenam A, Yuh B, Zhumkhawala A, et al. Prospective randomised non-inferiority trial of pelvic drain placement vs no pelvic drain placement after robot-assisted radical prostatectomy. BJU Int 2018;121:357–64.
31. Erlich T, Abu-Ghanem Y, Ramon J, et al. Postoperative urinary leakage following partial nephrectomy for renal mass: risk factors and a proposed algorithm for the diagnosis and management. Scand J Surg 2017;106:139–44.
32. Tachibana H, Iida S, Kondo T, et al. Possible impact of continuous drainage after minimally invasive partial nephrectomy. Int Urol Nephrol 2015;47:1763–9.
33. Kriegmair MC, Mandel P, Krombach P, et al. Drain placement can safely be omitted for open partial nephrectomy: results from a prospective randomized trial. Int J Urol 2016;23:390–4.
34. Tillier C, van Muilekom HAM, Bloos-van der Hulst J, et al. Vesico-urethral anastomosis (VUA) evaluation of short- and long-term outcome after robot-assisted laparoscopic radical prostatectomy (RARP): selective cystogram to improve outcome. J Robot Surg 2017;11:441–6.
35. Jian Z, Feng S, Chen Y, et al. Suprapubic tube versus urethral catheter drainage after robot-assisted radical prostatectomy: a systematic review and meta-analysis. BMC Urol 2018;18:1.

Enhanced Recovery After Surgery in Surgical Specialties
Gynecologic Oncology

Haller J. Smith, MD, Charles A. Leath III, MD, MSPH,
John Michael Straughn Jr, MD*

KEYWORDS

- Enhanced recovery after surgery • Gynecologic surgery • ERAS
- Surgical innovation

KEY POINTS

- Enhanced recovery after surgery has transformed perioperative care in gynecologic oncology and should be the standard of care.
- A multidisciplinary approach that includes input from gynecologic oncologists, anesthesia providers, and nursing staff is critical to successful protocol development.
- Institution-specific enhanced recovery after surgery goals should be developed to allow for auditing of compliance and monitoring of outcomes.

BACKGROUND

Founded as a nonprofit medical society in 2010, the Enhanced Recovery after Surgery (ERAS®) Society was the direct descendant of the ERAS Study Group that developed following an encounter at a nutritional symposium between Professors Ken Fearon and Olle Ljungqvist in 2001.[1] The goal of the ERAS Study Group was to examine what was known about ideal perioperative care and what was actually being performed in perioperative care. Ultimately, a mission statement was developed which focuses on 4 aspects of evidence-based practice: education, research, auditing, and implementation of evidence-based research to guide perioperative care decisions to improve outcomes.[1]

Much of the early work in ERAS was focused on its application in colorectal surgery. A Cochrane Review from 2011 evaluated the burgeoning field of ERAS in colorectal surgery and relied on 4 randomized, controlled trials that had been published and deemed acceptable for analysis.[2] In this early analysis, results from 237 patients were reported.

The authors have nothing to disclose.
Support: This research was supported in part by NIH-U10 CA180855 and 3P30CA013148-43S3 to C.A. Leath.
Division of Gynecologic Oncology, Department of Obstetrics and Gynecology, University of Alabama at Birmingham, 176F Room 10250, 619 19th Street South, Birmingham, AL 35249-7333, USA
* Corresponding author.
E-mail address: jstraughn@uabmc.edu

These studies demonstrated that although the level of available information was somewhat limited, ERAS patients had fewer complications (relative risk, 0.50; 95% confidence interval, 0.35–0.72), a shorter hospital duration of stay of approximately 2.94 days (95% confidence interval, −3.69 to −2.19), and comparable readmission rates.[2]

Before the ERAS® guidelines for gynecologic oncology were widely disseminated in 2016,[3,4] attention was being placed on the principles of ERAS even if the name itself was not used. One of the earliest publications of ERAS for gynecologic cancer surgery was from de Groot and colleagues[5] from the Netherlands. They evaluated the potential of spontaneous uptake of ERAS principals in a single institution when performed in other specialties. In this preintervention and postintervention study, they noted that although colorectal surgery was using an ERAS program, passive diffusion of these principles did not seem to spontaneously occur and suggested that a structured approach for gynecologic surgery was needed to maximize patient benefits.[5]

Following de Groot's publication, Nelson and colleagues[6] reported a systematic review of the published enhanced recovery pathways in an attempt to determine the current knowledge base as well as limitations in gynecologic cancer surgery. In this review, 7 heterogeneous trials generally included both a control group as well as an enhanced recovery group, although the largest study from Chase and colleagues[7] did not include a comparison arm. These trials evaluated preoperative, intraoperative, and postoperative factors that focused on preoperative education, avoidance of bowel preparation, multimodal analgesia, attention to fluid balance, early mobilization, diet and removal of drains, lines and catheters, and opioid restrictive analgesia. In summary, patients in the enhanced recovery pathways had a similar or shorter time to oral intake, shorter duration of stay, similar or fewer postoperative complications, similar or fewer reoperations, and less costly care. Importantly, these investigators noted that the auditing process as well as measuring compliance were key contributors to ensuring success of the program.[6]

Specific gynecologic oncologic surgical ERAS® recommendations were published in February 2016 and included 2 sets of guidelines: combined preoperative and intraoperative guidelines (Part I)[3] and a set of postoperative guidelines (Part II).[4] These extensive guidelines reviewed not only the specific areas of implementation in the entire perioperative process for gynecologic oncology surgery, but also incorporated the Grading of Recommendations, Assessment, Development and Evaluation (GRADE) system. The GRADE system reports not only an ordinal level of evidence from very low quality to high quality, with low and moderate quality in between, but also includes a binary recommendation strength of weak or strong. Importantly, although the level of evidence was variable, per the GRADE system for evaluated and reported guidelines, the majority of the evidence level was moderate or high quality, with all but 1 area having a strong recommendation grade. The highlights of the preoperative and intraoperative guidelines are presented in **Table 1**.

A separate publication from the same group reported on postoperative guidelines using the same approach and GRADE criteria.[4] As compared with the preoperative and intraoperative guidelines, the postoperative care guidelines are more varied in terms of their level of evidence and recommendation grades. Before ERAS®, interventions contrary to accepted surgical dogma, such as timing of feeding, use of drains, nasogastric compression and timing of urinary catheter removal, were starting to be evaluated and questioned.[4] Although many areas of postoperative management still need more study, a large number of the postoperative guidelines were still graded at a high level of evidence with a strong recommendation grade. **Table 2** provides the postoperative guidelines that meet both the high level of evidence and strong recommendation grade bar.

Table 1
Key enhanced recovery after surgery preoperative and intraoperative gynecologic oncology components with high level of evidence and a strong recommendation grade

Timing in Relationship to Surgery	Intervention
Preoperative	Smoking cessation 4 wk before surgery
Preoperative	Identify anemia preoperatively and correct before surgery
Preoperative	Allow clear liquids up to 2 h and solid food up to 6 h before surgery
Preoperative/ intraoperative	Patients at risk for VTE should receive both mechanical and pharmacologic prophylaxis
Preoperative	Oral contraceptive pill use should be discontinued before surgery and replaced with alternative form of contraception
Preoperative/ intraoperative	Prophylactic antibiotics should be administered within 60 min of skin incision with additional doses administered as needed for prolonged surgery and increased blood loss
Preoperative/ intraoperative	If needed, clipping hair is preferred over other methods
Preoperative/ intraoperative	Chlorhexidine-alcohol is the preferred skin preparation
Preoperative/ intraoperative	If appropriate with available resources and expertise, minimally invasive surgery is preferred
Intraoperative	Routine use of nasogastric decompression should be avoided
Intraoperative	Normothermia via the use of active warming devices
Intraoperative	Targeting euvolemia is preferred to either very liberal or restrictive fluid resuscitation

Abbreviation: VTE, venous thromboembolism.
Data from Nelson G, Altman AD, Nick A, et al. Guidelines for pre- and intra-operative care in gynecologic/oncology surgery: Enhanced Recovery After Surgery (ERAS®) Society recommendations–Part I. Gynecol Oncol 2016;140(2):313–22.

IMPLEMENTING AN ENHANCED RECOVERY AFTER SURGERY PROGRAM

With a wealth of available ERAS® information, including gynecologic oncology–specific guidelines,[3,6,8,9] the development of a new ERAS program at an institution still requires a dedicated and systematic approach.[5] Nelson and colleagues[9] have provided not only a framework including orders that may be used at each and every step, but additional commentary regarding each of the intervention issues that are part of the implementation process.

We believe that the development and implementation of any ERAS program, specifically a gynecologic oncology program, relies on the following principles: team implementation with an ERAS champion(s), project goals, institution-specific protocol development, and implementation of a database auditing both compliance and outcomes.

Before commencing with the development of a disease-specific ERAS program, a multispecialty team must be developed. This team should include anesthesia providers, gynecologic oncology surgeons, preoperative, and operating room and recovery room nurses, as well as both outpatient and inpatient nursing team members. Moreover, we designated champions that were responsible for leading the various parts of the team.

Before embarking on an ERAS program, goals need to be selected that are potentially obtainable as well as meaningful. In general, ERAS for gynecologic

Table 2
Key enhanced recovery after surgery postoperative gynecologic oncology components with high level of evidence and a strong recommendation grade

Aspect of Postoperative Care	Intervention
VTE prophylaxis	Well-fitted compression stockings and intermittent pneumatic compression should be used
VTE prophylaxis	Extending pharmacologic prophylaxis to 28 d should be used in patients undergoing a laparotomy for abdominal and/or pelvic malignancies
Nutrition	Resumption of a regular diet within 24 h of surgery is recommended
Nutrition/glycemic control	Mechanisms to reduce metabolic system should be enacted to decrease insulin resistance and hyperglycemia from developing
Nutrition/glycemic control	Perioperative maintenance of blood glucose <180–200 mg/dL is associated with ideal surgical outcomes
Analgesia	Multimodal analgesia should be used
Analgesia	NSAIDs and acetaminophen are preferred components of a multimodal approach
Analgesia	Thoracic epidural analgesia consisting of low-concentrations of local anesthetics with addition of opioids for up to 48 h can be considered

Abbreviations: NSAIDs, nonsteroidal antiinflammatory drug; VTE, venous thromboembolism.

Data from Nelson G, Altman AD, Nick A, et al. Guidelines for postoperative care in gynecologic/oncology surgery: Enhanced Recovery After Surgery (ERAS®) Society recommendations–Part II. Gynecol Oncol 2016;140(2):323–32.

surgery has attempted to decrease the hospital duration of stay, prevent preoperative catabolism with a quicker return to a postoperative diet, improve perioperative pain control, decrease reoperations and/or readmission, and improve the patient experience while decreasing costs.[6] Ideally, the electronic medical record system should be used and queried in such a manner that these data are automatically collected and collated. Importantly, these goals need strict definitions to allow successful auditing for both compliance and outcomes. When using the electronic medical record system, early review is important to ensure what is thought to be measured is in fact being measured and being measured accurately. Expertise in information technology is paramount to ensure accurate monitoring and measuring of program goals.

In addition to the development of ERAS program goals, protocol development is a laborious program that requires multiple reviews and revisions. With widespread adoption of ERAS programs at multiple institutions as well as freely available orders and review papers, the development of an internal protocol may be relatively straightforward. Nonetheless, this development still requires reviewing each aspect of the protocol from the initial patient encounter in the inpatient and/or outpatient setting, to hospital discharge and subsequent postoperative follow-up.

Following the development and implementation of an ERAS program is the auditing process. Auditing of the patient outcomes and for protocol compliance is necessary. When metrics are being correctly and adequately measured, areas that are below the prespecified thresholds are able to be identified and corrected. Correction may be necessary in either the performance of a certain aspect of the protocol, or in the documentation or capture of the element being performed. The original ERAS systems used an ERAS® Interactive Audit System.[6,10]

Using these principles, we identified relevant stakeholders and formed a core ERAS team. This team reviewed the ERAS® guidelines and published literature and determined which components would work best in our institution. The following section outlines the key components of our institutional protocol.

PREOPERATIVE COMPONENTS
Patient Education

One of the key components of a successful ERAS protocol is the implementation of comprehensive preoperative patient counseling and education. This step prepares the patient to take an active role in her recovery and sets realistic expectations for postoperative care, including duration of stay and postoperative pain control. This information should be provided in a manner that is easy to understand and, most important, all members of the perioperative care team should provide a consistent message. In our practice, patient education is initiated by the surgeon and reviewed in detail by the clinic nursing staff. Patients are provided with a booklet that introduces all members of the perioperative team, reviews preoperative and postdischarge instructions, and provides a day-by-day breakdown of what to expect during the postoperative hospital stay. This education is then reinforced by the anesthesia providers in the preoperative assessment, consultation, and treatment clinic and by the inpatient nursing staff.

Additionally, patients are emailed links to 2 educational videos, one that provides general information on gynecologic surgery and one that is specific to ERAS. Patients who do not have home computer access are given the opportunity to watch these videos in the clinic. Approximately 55% of our patients complete both videos in addition to the counseling they receive in clinic.

Preoperative Fluid Intake and Carbohydrate Loading

Despite recommendations to allow clear liquids up to 2 hours before surgery published by the American Society of Anesthesiologists in 1999, it has remained common practice to instruct patients to remain nothing by mouth after midnight before surgery.[11] In addition to dehydration, this strict fasting can also result in prolonged insulin resistance, which has been associated with hyperglycemia and increased postoperative complications. Preoperative carbohydrate loading can reverse this process and has other benefits, including improved patient satisfaction and decreased nausea.[12] We instruct patients to eat normally until midnight and then continue oral hydration with clear liquids until 2 hours before surgery. With the exception of poorly controlled diabetics, patients are also instructed to drink a carbohydrate-rich beverage, such as a sports drink, on their way to the hospital. This strategy ensures that patients receive a glucose load on the morning of surgery but does not result in any delay of their procedure because patients are instructed to arrive a minimum of 2 hours before surgery.

Preoperative Multimodal Analgesia

Preoperative multimodal analgesia has been shown to decrease pain scores and opioid requirements and decrease inflammation and stress response in patients undergoing gynecologic surgery.[13,14] Gabapentin also results in a significant decrease in postoperative nausea, pain, and opioid requirements in patients undergoing hysterectomy.[15] Although there are multiple acceptable regimens, our group elected to use a combination of acetaminophen, a nonsteroidal antiinflammatory drug, and gabapentin. Healthy patients with no contraindications are given acetaminophen 1000 mg, gabapentin 800 mg, and celecoxib 400 mg orally on arrival to the preoperative unit. These doses are decreased or held in elderly patients or those with impaired renal or hepatic function. Preoperative use of benzodiazepines and opioids is limited and avoided wherever possible.

INTRAOPERATIVE COMPONENTS
Maintenance of Normothermia

Intraoperative hypothermia has been associated with multiple adverse outcomes, including increased risk of wound infections, coagulopathy, and cardiovascular events.[3] We continuously monitor patients' body temperature intraoperatively using an esophageal probe and routinely use forced air warming blankets with a goal of maintaining body temperature of 96.8°F or higher.

Postoperative Nausea/Vomiting Prophylaxis

Patients are assessed at their preoperative assessment, consultation, and treatment visit for risk of developing postoperative nausea and vomiting using a standard algorithm and are subsequently stratified into low-, medium-, and high-risk categories. Low-risk patients are given ondansetron 4 mg intravenously (IV) 15 to 30 minutes before extubation. For medium-risk patients, dexamethasone 4 mg IV is added. High-risk patients receive both ondansetron and dexamethasone, have a scopolamine transdermal patch placed preoperatively, and are started on a continuous propofol infusion for all cases lasting longer than 1 hour.

Goal-Directed Fluid Resuscitation

One of the important tenets of ERAS is maintenance of euvolemia in the perioperative period.[3] To avoid intraoperative volume overload, we set basic parameters for fluid resuscitation in the operating room. Patients receive a base rate of 800 mL/h, which can be adjusted as needed to maintain adequate cardiac output. Normal saline is no longer used intraoperatively owing to the high salt load and has been replaced with lactated ringers or other isotonic solutions such as Plasma-Lyte. Hypotension may be treated with albumin or vasopressors as needed.

Nonopioid Adjuncts for Pain Control

All patients are given dexamethasone 0.1 mg/kg ideal body weight (maximum dose 8 mg) at the time of anesthesia induction to decrease inflammation and improve postoperative pain control. This dose can be decreased or held in patients with poorly controlled diabetes to avoid worsening postoperative hyperglycemia. Additionally, patients are treated with an intraoperative lidocaine infusion. Intraoperative use of opioids is largely avoided. If necessary, fentanyl is the opioid of choice owing to its short duration of action; morphine and hydromorphone are avoided.

Avoidance of Prophylactic Nasogastric Tubes

Historically, nasogastric tubes (NGTs) were frequently placed at the time of surgery in patients undergoing gynecologic surgery because they were thought to decrease postoperative ileus, reduce the risk of aspiration associated with postoperative vomiting, and prevent anastomotic leak. Evidence shows that NGTs actually increase the risk of pneumonia and do not decrease the risk of other complications. Additionally, they lead to increased duration of stay and patient discomfort.[16] Given these finding, we do not routinely place NGTs at the time of surgery, even if bowel resection is anticipated. If an NGT is placed for decompression intraoperatively, we recommend it be removed before the end of the procedure.

POSTOPERATIVE COMPONENTS
Postoperative Multimodal Analgesia

Similar to preoperative multimodal analgesia, the use of multimodal analgesia in the postoperative period has been associated with less pain and decreased opioid use. The combination of acetaminophen and nonsteroidal antiinflammatory drugs is particularly effective and has a greater effect than either agent given alone.[17] In our practice, healthy patients with acceptable renal and hepatic function are given scheduled acetaminophen beginning immediately postoperatively. For the first 24 hours postoperatively, they receive ketorolac 15 or 30 mg IV every 6 hours based on age, weight, and glomerular filtration rate and are subsequently transitioned to oral ibuprofen 200 to 600 mg every 6 hours. Patients who are unable to receive nonsteroidal antiinflammatory drugs for any reason are given tramadol 50 to 100 mg every 8 hours.

Regional analgesia is a critical part of the ERAS® protocol and can lead to significant opioid-sparing effects. Thoracic epidurals, intrathecal morphine injections, truncal nerve blocks such as the transversus abdominis plane block, or wound infiltration with local anesthetics have all been studied and found to have benefits.[4] Before the implementation of ERAS, we frequently used thoracic epidural analgesia for patients undergoing laparotomy. Although epidurals were effective for pain control, we found that they slowed postoperative mobility and prolonged the need for urinary catheters.[18] As a result, with the implementation of our ERAS protocol, we transitioned to intrathecal morphine injections as our regional analgesic of choice.

Unlike thoracic epidurals, intrathecal morphine injections do not hinder mobility, have a low risk of urinary retention, and are effective at decreasing postoperative pain for up to 48 hours.[19] Patients who are unable to receive intrathecal morphine owing to spinal hardware, coagulopathy, or other contraindications are offered a transversus abdominis plane block as an alternative. IV patient-controlled analgesia is reserved for patients who are unable to receive any regional analgesia. Less than 15% of patients have required patient-controlled analgesia for postoperative pain control since implementation of our ERAS protocol.

Although we have not used wound infiltration with local anesthetic in our protocol, other groups have found injection of long-acting local anesthetics such as liposomal bupivacaine to be effective at reducing postoperative opioid consumption in gynecologic oncology patients undergoing major surgery.[20] This step may be an effective alternative to the other types of regional analgesia described in this article.

Early Feeding

Traditionally, postoperative feeding protocols in gynecology patients included gradual advancement from nothing by mouth to a liquid diet, and a regular diet was only provided once a patient had evidence of return of bowel function. This gradual reintroduction of oral intake stemmed from the fear that early feeding would increase the incidence of postoperative complications such as ileus or wound complications; however, this practice was not evidence based.[21] In fact, there are a substantial data that suggests that, although early feeding may increase the incidence of early postoperative nausea, it does not increase rates of ileus or pulmonary complications and actually decreases risks of infectious complications and duration of stay.[16,22–24] Thus, advancement to a regular diet is recommended within 24 hours of surgery for gynecologic surgery patients.[4] In our practice, patients are allowed to have liquids immediately postoperatively and are advanced to a regular diet as tolerated within the first 24 hours. They are provided with nutritional shakes at each meal to supplement their caloric intake in the early postoperative period. Additionally, patients are encouraged to chew gum postoperatively because there is some evidence that this may accelerate the return of bowel function.[25,26]

Maintenance of Euvolemia

Given recommendations for early feeding, most patients do not require IV hydration for longer than 24 hours postoperatively.[4] In addition to IV poles limiting mobility,[27] fluid overload can result in pulmonary edema, increased risk of ileus, and a prolonged duration of stay.[8] Our ERAS patients are started on lactated ringers at 40 mL/h in the immediate postoperative period, which can be increased if needed for suspected hypovolemia. Fluid boluses are restricted to use in patients with hemodynamic evidence of hypovolemia or profound oliguria. IV fluids are discontinued early on the morning of postoperative day 1 in all patients who are tolerating liquids orally.

Early Mobility

The benefits of early postoperative ambulation include decreased pulmonary complications, less muscle atrophy, and prevention of thromboembolic complications.[4] We provide our patients with a structured plan for postoperative mobility, which is initially discussed during their preoperative counseling and reinforced postoperatively. Patients are expected to ambulate in the room and get out of bed to a chair on the day of surgery. From postoperative day 1 through the day of discharge, they are expected to be out of bed for at least 8 hours a day and ambulate in the hall 4 times daily.

Early Foley Catheter Removal

Prolonged use of a urinary catheter after hysterectomy has been associated with increased risk of urinary tract infection and decreased ambulation; therefore, urinary catheter removal is recommended at less than 24 hours postoperatively as part of ERAS protocols.[4,27] Unless patients have a bladder injury requiring prolonged catheter drainage, we routinely remove urinary catheters on the morning of postoperative day 1.

Discharge Planning

Discharge planning begins on postoperative day 1 with anticipation of discharge on postoperative day 2 in the majority of patients. Nurses are required to document daily weights, patient showers, and ambulation. Patients are discharged when they are tolerating a diet, voiding, and have adequate pain control. A review of the patient's narcotic history and postoperative use is performed at the time of discharge and a narcotic prescription is provided. Lovenox is prescribed for 21 days for patients with a cancer diagnosis or if they are at high risk for clotting. All patients receive an automated phone call with 72 hours of discharge to assess for postoperative issues or complications. Patients are provided a postoperative appointment with their surgeon within 28 days of discharge.

OUTCOMES IN GYNECOLOGIC ONCOLOGY

ERAS protocols have become more refined and recent evidence suggests that patient outcomes are improved and opioid use is decreased. Modesitt and colleagues[28] developed 2 different ERAS protocols for their gynecologic oncology patients that used components of preoperative, intraoperative, and postoperative ERAS care—a full ERAS pathway using regional anesthesia for open procedures and a light ERAS pathway without regional anesthesia for patients undergoing vaginal and minimally invasive surgery. A before-and-after study design compared clinical outcomes, costs, and patient satisfaction. In the full ERAS protocol, 136 patients were compared with 211 historical controls. The median duration of stay was reduced (2.0 vs 3.0 days; $P = .007$) as well as total complications (21.3% vs 40.2%; $P = .004$). Reductions were seen in median intraoperative morphine equivalents (0.3 vs 12.7 mg; $P<.001$) and immediate postoperative pain scores (3.7 vs 5.0; $P<.001$). These investigators concluded that implementation of ERAS protocols in gynecologic surgery was associated with a substantial decrease in morphine administration, reduction in duration of stay for open procedures, improved patient satisfaction, and decreased hospital costs.[28]

In 2017, Dickson and colleagues[29] published their results from a prospective, randomized, controlled trial comparing an ERAS protocol with routine postoperative care in women undergoing laparotomy on a gynecologic oncology service. A sample size of 50 per group was planned to achieve 80% power to detect a 2-day difference in duration of stay (decrease from 5 to 3 days). There were 103 eligible patients who were enrolled, 52 in the control group and 51 in the ERAS group. Interestingly, the investigators found no difference in duration of stay between the 2 groups (median 3.0 days in both groups; $P = .36$). ERAS patients used less narcotics on day 0 (10.0 morphine equivalents vs 5.5 morphine equivalents; $P = .09$) and day 2 (10.0 morphine equivalents vs 7.5 morphine equivalents; $P = .05$). The authors reported no difference in ambulation, gastrointestinal issues, complications, or readmissions in the 2 groups, and concluded that introducing a formal ERAS protocol did not significantly improve outcomes.[29] Critics have concluded that this was a poorly defined prospective trial, because few ERAS elements were implemented, compliance was not measured, and the use of ERAS tenets likely occurred in the control arm.

We initiated our ERAS program at the University of Alabama at Birmingham in November 2016, which includes all patients undergoing elective laparotomy. In the first 13 months, 213 patients were enrolled. We initially had monthly audit meetings to review data from an institutional financial database as well as ERAS-specific tracking board that imports both compliance and outcome metrics directly from the electronic medical record. After 6 months, we transitioned to quarterly meetings with the other ERAS programs including colorectal and urology. Since the initiation of our gynecologic oncology protocol, our observed to expected duration of stay index has been reduced to less than 0.82, and monthly readmissions have been less than 6%, except for 4 months. Compliance and documentation has been excellent with ambulation, regular diet, deep venous thrombosis prophylaxis, multimodal analgesia, and the use of blocks.

We performed a retrospective cohort study at University of Alabama at Birmingham evaluating the impact of an ERAS protocol on pain control in gynecologic oncology patients undergoing elective laparotomy. ERAS patients were compared with a control group from the year before ERAS implementation. Although ERAS significantly reduced postoperative pain scores and the amount of narcotics required at discharge in narcotic-naïve patients, there was no difference in either outcome in the chronic narcotic users. Despite a lack of significant improvement in postoperative pain in chronic narcotic users, ERAS still had benefits in this population, including decreased duration of stay.[30]

SUMMARY

Emerging data suggest that ERAS should be the standard of care for gynecologic oncology patients undergoing major abdominal surgery. Similar ERAS components can be used to improve patient well-being and satisfaction in patients undergoing minimally invasive surgery. With the growing visibility and focus on the opioid crisis in the United States, patients are more receptive to avoiding postoperative narcotics that may lead to dependence or abuse. Implementation of ERAS protocols can help us to provide opioid-free recovery to many of our patients.

REFERENCES

1. ERAS Society. Available at: http://erassociety.org/about/history/. Accessed February 25, 2018.
2. Spanjersberg WR, Reurings J, Keus F, et al. Fast track surgery versus conventional recovery strategies for colorectal surgery. Cochrane Database Syst Rev 2011;(2):CD007635.
3. Nelson G, Altman AD, Nick A, et al. Guidelines for pre- and intra-operative care in gynecologic/oncology surgery: Enhanced Recovery After Surgery (ERAS(R)) Society recommendations–Part I. Gynecol Oncol 2016;140(2):313–22.
4. Nelson G, Altman AD, Nick A, et al. Guidelines for postoperative care in gynecologic/oncology surgery: Enhanced Recovery After Surgery (ERAS(R)) Society recommendations–Part II. Gynecol Oncol 2016;140(2):323–32.
5. de Groot JJ, van Es LE, Maessen JM, et al. Diffusion of Enhanced Recovery principles in gynecologic oncology surgery: is active implementation still necessary? Gynecol Oncol 2014;134(3):570–5.
6. Nelson G, Kalogera E, Dowdy SC. Enhanced recovery pathways in gynecologic oncology. Gynecol Oncol 2014;135(3):586–94.
7. Chase DM, Lopez S, Nguyen C, et al. A clinical pathway for postoperative management and early patient discharge: does it work in gynecologic oncology? Am J Obstet Gynecol 2008;199(5):541.e1-7.
8. Kalogera E, Dowdy SC. Enhanced recovery pathway in gynecologic surgery: improving outcomes through evidence-based medicine. Obstet Gynecol Clin North Am 2016;43(3):551–73.
9. Nelson G, Dowdy SC, Lasala J, et al. Enhanced recovery after surgery (ERAS(R)) in gynecologic oncology - Practical considerations for program development. Gynecol Oncol 2017;147(3):617–20.
10. ERAS Interactive Audit System (EIAS). 2014. Available at: http://www.erassociety.org/index.php/eras-care-system/eras-interactive-audit-system. Accessed February 25, 2018.
11. Practice guidelines for preoperative fasting and the use of pharmacologic agents to reduce the risk of pulmonary aspiration: application to healthy patients undergoing elective procedures: a report by the American Society of Anesthesiologist Task Force on Preoperative Fasting. Anesthesiology 1999; 90(3):896–905.
12. Sarin A, Chen LL, Wick EC. Enhanced recovery after surgery-Preoperative fasting and glucose loading-A review. J Surg Oncol 2017;116(5):578–82.
13. Chen JQ, Wu Z, Wen LY, et al. Preoperative and postoperative analgesic techniques in the treatment of patients undergoing transabdominal hysterectomy: a preliminary randomized trial. BMC Anesthesiol 2015;15:70.
14. Steinberg AC, Schimpf MO, White AB, et al. Preemptive analgesia for postoperative hysterectomy pain control: systematic review and clinical practice guidelines. Am J Obstet Gynecol 2017;217(3):303–13.e6.
15. Alayed N, Alghanaim N, Tan X, et al. Preemptive use of gabapentin in abdominal hysterectomy: a systematic review and meta-analysis. Obstet Gynecol 2014; 123(6):1221–9.

16. Fanning J, Valea FA. Perioperative bowel management for gynecologic surgery. Am J Obstet Gynecol 2011;205(4):309–14.
17. Ong CK, Seymour RA, Lirk P, et al. Combining paracetamol (acetaminophen) with nonsteroidal antiinflammatory drugs: a qualitative systematic review of analgesic efficacy for acute postoperative pain. Anesth Analg 2010;110(4):1170–9.
18. Chen LM, Weinberg VK, Chen C, et al. Perioperative outcomes comparing patient controlled epidural versus intravenous analgesia in gynecologic oncology surgery. Gynecol Oncol 2009;115(3):357–61.
19. Levy BF, Scott MJ, Fawcett W, et al. Randomized clinical trial of epidural, spinal or patient-controlled analgesia for patients undergoing laparoscopic colorectal surgery. Br J Surg 2011;98(8):1068–78.
20. Kalogera E, Bakkum-Gamez JN, Weaver AL, et al. Abdominal incision injection of liposomal bupivacaine and opioid use after laparotomy for gynecologic malignancies. Obstet Gynecol 2016;128(5):1009–17.
21. Fanning J, Andrews S. Early postoperative feeding after major gynecologic surgery: evidence-based scientific medicine. Am J Obstet Gynecol 2001;185(1):1–4.
22. Charoenkwan K, Matovinovic E. Early versus delayed oral fluids and food for reducing complications after major abdominal gynaecologic surgery. Cochrane Database Syst Rev 2014;(12):CD004508.
23. Pearl ML, Valea FA, Fischer M, et al. A randomized controlled trial of early postoperative feeding in gynecologic oncology patients undergoing intra-abdominal surgery. Obstet Gynecol 1998;92(1):94–7.
24. Schilder JM, Hurteau JA, Look KY, et al. A prospective controlled trial of early postoperative oral intake following major abdominal gynecologic surgery. Gynecol Oncol 1997;67(3):235–40.
25. Pereira Gomes Morais E, Riera R, Porfírio GJ, et al. Chewing gum for enhancing early recovery of bowel function after caesarean section. Cochrane Database Syst Rev 2016;(10):CD011562.
26. Mei B, Wang W, Cui F, et al. Chewing gum for intestinal function recovery after colorectal cancer surgery: a systematic review and meta-analysis. Gastroenterol Res Pract 2017;2017:3087904.
27. Liebermann M, Awad M, Dejong M, et al. Ambulation of hospitalized gynecologic surgical patients: a randomized controlled trial. Obstet Gynecol 2013;121(3):533–7.
28. Modesitt SC, Sarosiek BM, Trowbridge ER, et al. Enhanced recovery implementation in major gynecologic surgeries: effect of care standardization. Obstet Gynecol 2016;128(3):457–66.
29. Dickson EL, Stockwell E, Geller MA, et al. Enhanced recovery program and length of stay after laparotomy on a gynecologic oncology service: a randomized controlled trial. Obstet Gynecol 2017;129(2):355–62.
30. Smith HJ, Boitano TL, Leath CA III, et al. Impact of ERAS on postoperative pain control in chronic narcotic users. Presented at the Society of Gynecologic Oncology Annual Meeting on Women's Cancer, New Orleans, LA 2018.

Enhanced Recovery After Surgery and Future Directions

Amit Merchea, MD[a],*, David W. Larson, MD, MBA[b]

KEYWORDS

- ERAS • ERP • Enhanced recovery • Prehabilitation • Perioperative surgical home
- Telemedicine

KEY POINTS

- Although utilization of enhanced recovery after surgery (ERAS) protocols is becoming more mainstream and greater numbers of specialties are beginning to consider it standard of care, there must be an ongoing focus on compliance and the entire perioperative period.
- This is particularly important because ERAS, by practice, shifts much of the perioperative care to outside the hospital.
- Whatever methods are used, the underlying goal should be the same—to provide high-value, evidence-based care.

INTRODUCTION

Since the concept of enhanced recovery after surgery (ERAS) was first published by Henrik Kehlet in the late 1990s,[1] the adoption and dissemination of these pathways have proved clinically and financially beneficial.[2–4] The underlying goal of these pathways has persisted—an attempt to maintain surgical patients in a physiologically normal state by minimizing the effects of surgical stress. These efforts reside in 3 distinct, but interconnected, phases—the preoperative phase, the intraoperative phase, and the postoperative phase.

Despite broad diffusion of ERAS protocol across numerous specialties, barriers to implementation and achieving high compliance remain a challenge.[5,6] As protocols have become more complicated, implementation has been further delayed secondary to organizational and provider-specific factors.[7] Interventions and processes to improve compliance, eliminate barriers, and to better integrate the phases of care

The authors have nothing to disclose.
[a] Division of Colon and Rectal Surgery, Mayo Clinic, Mayo Clinic College of Medicine, 4500 San Pablo Road, Jacksonville, FL 32224, USA; [b] Division of Colon and Rectal Surgery, Mayo Clinic, 200 First Street SW, Rochester, MN, 55905, USA
* Corresponding author.
E-mail address: Merchea.Amit@mayo.edu

ultimately form the focus of the future directions of ERAS. In the authors' opinion, central components of this include the maintenance of the core tenets of ERAS across specialties (opioid avoidance, euvolemia, early mobilization, early feeding, and so forth), development of prehabilitation programs, implementation of the surgical home, and use of novel technology for reporting outcomes.

PROLIFERATION ACROSS SPECIALTIES

Colorectal surgery was among the first specialties to implement ERAS pathways. Since the early 2000s, most major specialties have instituted some form of accelerated recovery pathway with evidence-based specialty-specific interventions. These have included gynecology/gynecologic oncology, urology, bariatrics/foregut, orthopedics, and others.[8–14]

Although the fundamentals and basic elements of ERAS are consistent across specialties, the specialty-specific interventions (for example, limitation of drain placement in pancreaticoduodenectomy, preoperative weight loss goals in bariatrics, novel analgesic/anesthetic use in orthopedics, and preoperative respiratory physiotherapy in thoracic surgery) may improve specific outcome measures within those specialties.[15] There is debate, however, whether these increasingly complex protocols ultimately lead to delayed implementation and lack of compliance.[7] Furthermore, limited data exist regarding the impact, contribution, and compliance of individual elements within these increasingly complex protocols.[16]

As further dissemination of ERAS occurs, it will become increasingly necessary to focus implementation strategies on already recognized and scientifically established practices. This would further address the knowing-doing gap, previously described by Kehlet.[7] Kehlet further contends that as new interventions and technologies are used within innovative ERAS protocols, future research efforts must include the current knowledge and base of evidence.[16,17]

PREHABILITATION

The focus on physical conditioning has largely been in the postoperative recovery period. Limitations in patient preoperative functional/physical capacity, however, have been shown to increase postoperative morbidity and mortality and lengthen overall recovery.[18] This is particularly true in the cancer patient population, where neoadjuvant therapies may lead to further declines in fitness and performance status.[19] Prehabilitation is the process that has been proposed to preemptively improve functional and psychological capacity and promote postoperative recovery. Three main pillars of prehabilitation are exercise, nutrition, and psychological stress reduction. The desired effects of such pathways are complementary to ERAS and may serve to improve many shared outcomes. High-level data in this arena, however, are conflicting.

Among the earliest reviews was one published by Valkenet and colleagues[20] that included 12 studies reviewing the effect of preoperative exercise on postoperative complications in cardiac, orthopedic, and abdominal vascular surgery. This study demonstrated that preoperative exercise was correlated with reduced postoperative complications and earlier discharge in those undergoing cardiac and abdominal surgery but not in those undergoing orthopedic surgery.

Lemanu and colleagues[21] performed another systematic review reviewing similar operative procedures and found that there was little evidence of clinical improvement in the setting of poor adherence to the prescribed interventions. This group conceded the heterogeneity and lack of adherence as possible factors in the negative findings. Conversely, a study looking specifically at total body prehabilitation (targeting of systemic musculoskeletal and cardiovascular deconditioning) reviewed 21 studies and found improvements in postoperative pain, length of stay, and functional capacity. Issues of study heterogeneity and quality, however, remained a recognized bias.[22]

Several recent randomized trials have also been published on this subject. Gillis and colleagues[23] described a multimodal program of exercise, nutritional counseling with protein supplementation, and relaxation exercises as part of a prehabilitation cohort and compared this with a standard rehabilitation group. This trial reported an increased walking capacity preoperatively and that a significant proportion of patients were at or above baseline exercise capacity at 8 weeks postoperatively (84 vs 62%; $P = .049$) in the prehabilitation cohort.

Overall evidence for prehabilitation is in its infancy and definitive recommendations regarding the implementation of prehabilitation as part of a larger ERAS program are difficult to make based on the extant literature. It seems reasonable, however, to conclude that prehabilitation shares many goals and overlaps with ERAS. The combination of interventions (prehabilitation within a defined ERAS pathway) may prove to have a greater effect than either individually.[24] Future research, the authors believe, should be directed toward investigating this and other surgery-specific prehabilitation interventions.

THE PERIOPERATIVE SURGICAL HOME

The concept of the perioperative surgical home (PSH) was developed in response to high costs and variable quality of health care. The main tenets of the PSH are to improve the patient experience, improve the overall quality of care, and reduce costs. Although ERAS functions within the immediate preoperative, intraoperative, and postoperative periods, the PSH serves to broaden the overall phases of care, promote a team-based multidisciplinary system, and complement the ERAS pathway.[25] It has further been argued that given the relatively slow uptake of ERAS and inconsistent compliance of its elements, an ERAS protocol in isolation may be insufficient to produce sustained improvements in patient care.[26]

There is a paucity of data on the use of a PSH and further study is necessary on this patient-centric approach. The growing role of accountable care organizations, pay-for-performance, and bundled payments puts further pressure on achieving high-value care (high quality and low cost) in nonintegrated health care systems.[27] This high-value care extends beyond the immediate perioperative period impacted by ERAS and includes the expanded areas that a PSH would affect. This seems particularly true given that ERAS pathways have shifted much of patient convalescence from an in-hospital setting to an external outpatient setting. It remains to be seen if the adoption of a PSH will become more commonplace as these health care economics pressures increase.

TECHNOLOGY IN FOLLOW-UP AND PATIENT OUTCOMES

Numerous technological devices have emerged since the development of ERAS and may facilitate patient recovery and reporting. Advancements in computing and the ubiquitous nature of smart devices have created the possibility of telemedicine for postoperative follow-up and the use of wearable devices to monitor and report patient outcomes.[15,28] These advancements also have the potential to have an impact on the preoperative period by enhancing access to healthcare and bringing specialty care to regions that may otherwise be lacking.[29]

A recent meta-analysis on telemedicine postdischarge revealed that such processes were safe, effective, and economically beneficial. All included studies were hampered, however, by small sample sizes and significant selection bias, and most studies have been in the ambulatory or low-risk setting.[30]

Katz and colleagues[31] reported their experience with a prospective teledischarge program, in which patients undergoing pancreatectomy had 2 virtual visits postoperatively. A majority of patients (80%) believed their postoperative care was "enhanced" by the virtual visits and approximately 30% of patients had some intervention completed given findings at the time of the virtual visit.

Martinez-Ramos and colleagues[32] investigated the use of mobile phone–based telemedicine to transmit postoperative images to the care team. They found that approximately 70% of patients had their concerns adequately addressed based on review of images alone and fewer than 5% of patients were asked to return to the hospital earlier than planned. This group concluded that telemedicine improved the efficiency of outpatient follow-up and avoided unnecessary hospital visits. Recently, Pecorelli and colleagues[28] published their results of a pilot study assessing the validity and usability of a mobile application for patient education and self-reporting. In their study of 45 patients, completion rates of the prescribed queries were high (89%) and a majority of patients (89%) found it helped in some manner in their recovery. Their novel approach, reported success, and usability underscore the opportunities that exist with further development of such technologies. Further efforts with such mobile applications should be directed toward improving pathway compliance and providing continuous feedback to providers.

Other groups have considered the use of wearable sensors/devices to monitor physical activity postoperatively.[33] Widespread adoption and integration of such wearable devices are limited despite advances in the reported variables (including vital signs and extent of body movement). The potential benefits, however, to the clinician are significant by providing patient data to monitor recovery and identify those needing intervention.[34]

The use of technology in the form of telemedicine or wearable sensors can serve to complement ERAS in many ways. In the preoperative phase, data can be gathered regarding patient activity and can identify potential patients at risk of needing greater postoperative care. The ability to capture in-hospital, postoperative data may aide in discharge decision making and planning. Finally, use of novel patient interaction tools may facilitate postoperative evaluation.

SUMMARY

In summary, although use of ERAS protocols is becoming more mainstream and greater numbers of specialties are beginning to consider it standard of care, there must be an ongoing focus on compliance and the entire perioperative period. This is particularly important because ERAS, by practice, shifts much of the perioperative care to outside the hospital. Whatever methods are used, the underlying goal should be the same—to provide high-value, evidence-based care. Ultimately, this can only facilitate what Kehlet and Joshi[17] described as the overall aim of ERAS—that is, achieving a "risk and pain free operation."

REFERENCES

1. Kehlet H. Multimodal approach to control postoperative pathophysiology and rehabilitation. Br J Anaesth 1997;78(5):606–17.
2. Kehlet H, Wilmore DW. Evidence-based surgical care and the evolution of fast-track surgery. Ann Surg 2008;248(2):189–98.

3. Ljungqvist O, Scott M, Fearon KC. Enhanced recovery after surgery: a review. JAMA Surg 2017;152(3):292–8.

4. Larson DW, Lovely JK, Cima RR, et al. Outcomes after implementation of a multi-modal standard care pathway for laparoscopic colorectal surgery. Br J Surg 2014;101(8):1023–30.

5. McLeod RS, Aarts MA, Chung F, et al. Development of an enhanced recovery after surgery guideline and implementation strategy based on the knowledge-to-action cycle. Ann Surg 2015;262(6):1016–25.

6. ERAS Compliance Group. The impact of enhanced recovery protocol compliance on elective colorectal cancer resection: results from an international registry. Ann Surg 2015;261(6):1153–9.

7. Kehlet H. Enhanced Recovery After Surgery (ERAS): good for now, but what about the future? Can J Anaesth 2015;62(2):99–104.

8. Nelson G, Altman AD, Nick A, et al. Guidelines for pre- and intra-operative care in gynecologic/oncology surgery: Enhanced Recovery After Surgery (ERAS(R)) Society recommendations–Part I. Gynecol Oncol 2016;140(2):313–22.

9. Nelson G, Altman AD, Nick A, et al. Guidelines for postoperative care in gynecologic/oncology surgery: Enhanced Recovery After Surgery (ERAS(R)) Society recommendations–Part II. Gynecol Oncol 2016;140(2):323–32.

10. Cerantola Y, Valerio M, Persson B, et al. Guidelines for perioperative care after radical cystectomy for bladder cancer: Enhanced Recovery After Surgery (ERAS((R))) society recommendations. Clin Nutr 2013;32(6):879–87.

11. Lassen K, Coolsen MM, Slim K, et al. Guidelines for perioperative care for pancreaticoduodenectomy: Enhanced Recovery After Surgery (ERAS(R)) Society recommendations. World J Surg 2013;37(2):240–58.

12. Lemanu DP, Srinivasa S, Singh PP, et al. Optimizing perioperative care in bariatric surgery patients. Obes Surg 2012;22(6):979–90.

13. Jones NL, Edmonds L, Ghosh S, et al. A review of enhanced recovery for thoracic anaesthesia and surgery. Anaesthesia 2013;68(2):179–89.

14. Ibrahim MS, Twaij H, Giebaly DE, et al. Enhanced recovery in total hip replacement: a clinical review. Bone Joint J 2013;95-B(12):1587–94.

15. Abeles A, Kwasnicki RM, Darzi A. Enhanced recovery after surgery: current research insights and future direction. World J Gastrointest Surg 2017;9(2):37–45.

16. Slim K, Kehlet H. Commentary: fast track surgery: the need for improved study design. Colorectal Dis 2012;14(8):1013–4.

17. Kehlet H, Joshi GP. Enhanced recovery after surgery: current controversies and concerns. Anesth Analg 2017;125(6):2154–5.

18. Wilson RJ, Davies S, Yates D, et al. Impaired functional capacity is associated with all-cause mortality after major elective intra-abdominal surgery. Br J Anaesth 2010;105(3):297–303.

19. West MA, Loughney L, Lythgoe D, et al. Effect of prehabilitation on objectively measured physical fitness after neoadjuvant treatment in preoperative rectal cancer patients: a blinded interventional pilot study. Br J Anaesth 2015;114(2):244–51.

20. Valkenet K, van de Port IG, Dronkers JJ, et al. The effects of preoperative exercise therapy on postoperative outcome: a systematic review. Clin Rehabil 2011;25(2):99–111.

21. Lemanu DP, Singh PP, MacCormick AD, et al. Effect of preoperative exercise on cardiorespiratory function and recovery after surgery: a systematic review. World J Surg 2013;37(4):711–20.

22. Santa Mina D, Clarke H, Ritvo P, et al. Effect of total-body prehabilitation on post-operative outcomes: a systematic review and meta-analysis. Physiotherapy 2014; 100(3):196–207.
23. Gillis C, Li C, Lee L, et al. Prehabilitation versus rehabilitation: a randomized control trial in patients undergoing colorectal resection for cancer. Anesthesiology 2014;121(5):937–47.
24. Carli F, Silver JK, Feldman LS, et al. Surgical prehabilitation in patients with cancer: state-of-the-science and recommendations for future research from a panel of subject matter experts. Phys Med Rehabil Clin N Am 2017;28(1):49–64.
25. King AB, Alvis BD, McEvoy MD. Enhanced recovery after surgery, perioperative medicine, and the perioperative surgical home: current state and future implications for education and training. Curr Opin Anaesthesiol 2016;29(6):727–32.
26. Pearsall EA, Meghji Z, Pitzul KB, et al. A qualitative study to understand the barriers and enablers in implementing an enhanced recovery after surgery program. Ann Surg 2015;261(1):92–6.
27. Desebbe O, Lanz T, Kain Z, et al. The perioperative surgical home: an innovative, patient-centred and cost-effective perioperative care model. Anaesth Crit Care Pain Med 2016;35(1):59–66.
28. Pecorelli N, Fiore JF Jr, Kaneva P, et al. An app for patient education and self-audit within an enhanced recovery program for bowel surgery: a pilot study assessing validity and usability. Surg Endosc 2018;32(5):2263–73.
29. Canon S, Shera A, Patel A, et al. A pilot study of telemedicine for post-operative urological care in children. J Telemed Telecare 2014;20(8):427–30.
30. Gunter RL, Chouinard S, Fernandes-Taylor S, et al. Current use of telemedicine for post-discharge surgical care: a systematic review. J Am Coll Surg 2016; 222(5):915–27.
31. Katz MH, Slack R, Bruno M, et al. Outpatient virtual clinical encounters after complex surgery for cancer: a prospective pilot study of "TeleDischarge". J Surg Res 2016;202(1):196–203.
32. Martinez-Ramos C, Cerdan MT, Lopez RS. Mobile phone-based telemedicine system for the home follow-up of patients undergoing ambulatory surgery. Telemed J E Health 2009;15(6):531–7.
33. Appelboom G, Camacho E, Abraham ME, et al. Smart wearable body sensors for patient self-assessment and monitoring. Arch Public Health 2014;72(1):28.
34. Appelboom G, Yang AH, Christophe BR, et al. The promise of wearable activity sensors to define patient recovery. J Clin Neurosci 2014;21(7):1089–93.

Moving?

Make sure your subscription moves with you!

To notify us of your new address, find your **Clinics Account Number** (located on your mailing label above your name), and contact customer service at:

Email: journalscustomerservice-usa@elsevier.com

800-654-2452 (subscribers in the U.S. & Canada)
314-447-8871 (subscribers outside of the U.S. & Canada)

Fax number: 314-447-8029

Elsevier Health Sciences Division
Subscription Customer Service
3251 Riverport Lane
Maryland Heights, MO 63043

*To ensure uninterrupted delivery of your subscription, please notify us at least 4 weeks in advance of move.

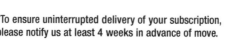